A TATTOO ON MY BRAIN

Dr Daniel Gibbs is one of 50 million people worldwide with an Alzheimer's disease diagnosis. Unlike most patients with Alzheimer's, however, Dr Gibbs worked as a neurologist for twenty-five years, caring for patients with the very disease now affecting him. Also unusual is that Dr Gibbs had begun to suspect he had Alzheimer's several years before any official diagnosis could be made. Forewarned by genetic testing showing he carried alleles that increased the risk of developing the disease, he noticed symptoms of mild cognitive impairment long before any tests would have alerted him. In this highly personal account, Dr Gibbs documents the effect his diagnosis has had on his life and explains his advocacy for improving early recognition of Alzheimer's. Weaving clinical knowledge from decades caring for dementia patients with his personal experience of the disease, this is an optimistic tale of one man's journey with early-stage Alzheimer's disease.

Daniel Gibbs is a retired neurologist in Portland, Oregon with early-stage Alzheimer's disease. Having spent twenty-five years caring for patients, many with dementia themselves, he is now an active advocate for the early recognition and management of Alzheimer's.

Teresa H. Barker is journalist and nonfiction book cowriter whose collaborations include strong narrative treatments of subjects including medical science, creative aging, child and adult development, parenting and life in the digital age.

"The patient perspective in Alzheimer's is often sorely missing from international dialogue and debate about this demon disease. Dr. Daniel Gibbs, whom I am honored to call a friend in this journey, has connected the serpentine dots between the patient and the medical profession in his brilliant work, A Tattoo on my Brain. As a retired neurologist and now a patient, Dr. Gibbs writes with great passion, knowledge and perseverance. His resolve reminds me of William Ernest Henley's poem Invictus: 'My head is bloody, but unbowed.' A Tattoo on My Brain is a must read for the world."

Greg O'Brien, author of On Pluto: Inside the Mind of Alzheimer's

"As a neurologist with early-stage Alzheimer's, Dr. Daniel Gibbs offers a uniquely insightful, candid, and compassionate view from both seats. A Tattoo on My Brain is essential reading for any family living with an Alzheimer's diagnosis."

Lisa Genova, New York Times bestselling author of Still Alice and Remember: The Science of Memory and the Art of Forgetting

"When a neurologist experiences a so-called neurodegenerative condition such as Alzheimer's or Parkinson disease they are often equipped uniquely to provide insight into a condition that non-medically qualified patients may lack. In this unique work, A Tattoo on My Brain, Dr. Gibbs tracks in meticulous detail the earliest symptoms of what was diagnosed subsequently as Alzheimer's disease. Interestingly, the apparent prodromal symptom was smell impairment appearing some 10 years before diagnosis of AD although that could have related in part to a coincidental pituitary adenoma. Either way, smell loss is now a well-recognised feature of AD and in Dr. Gibbs' case, the insidious decline of smell appreciation is evaluated by serial measurement on the University of Pennsylvania Smell Identification Test. The possibility of late onset AD did not come as a complete surprise, given that he was a homozygous carrier for the APOE-4 allele. Subsequent impairment of declarative memory with abnormalities on amyloid PET imaging put the diagnosis beyond reasonable doubt. Dr. Gibbs comments on the role of cholinesterase and glutamate antagonists and describes his unfortunate experience with aducanumab, the monoclonal antibody against amyloid. Finally, the role of lifestyle and dietary changes are discussed as a means to retard the progress of the disease. This work will have major appeal to lay people, especially those caring for an affected family member but also to neurologists, neuropsychologists and those involved in trials of new medications."

Professor Christopher H Hawkes, MD, FRCP, FAAN, Honorary Professor of Neurology, Barts School of Medicine & Dentistry, Honorary Consultant Neurologist, Barts Health, Author of Smell and Taste Disorders

"Dr. Gibbs provides a first-hand account of his journey as a neurologist living with early-stage Alzheimer's that is thoughtful, educational, humorous and poignant. I highly recommend this book to patients and families living with Alzheimer's, and to doctors and scientists dedicated to studying the disease and developing new therapies."

Gil Rabinovici, MD, Professor of Neurology, University of California San Francisco

"*A Tattoo on My Brain* describes Dr. Daniel Gibbs' amazing journey from neurologist to patient living with Alzheimer's disease. Clues crop up along the way, a genetic marker for Alzheimer's, strange odors and memory glitches that tipped him off that his brain was starting to malfunction. He underwent advanced brain scans that showed the buildup of amyloid plaques and he joined a clinical trial to remove them. He vividly describes the side effects that briefly turned his world upside down. But Dr. Gibbs emerges from this odyssey in good shape, with wisdom and reflection urging readers to learn about their risk for Alzheimer's disease and take steps to prevent it."

Stephen Salloway, MD, MS, Director of Neurology and the Memory and Aging Program, Butler Hospital, Providence, Rhode Island, and Martin M. Zucker Professor of Psychiatry and Human Behavior and Professor of Neurology, Warren Alpert Medical School of Brown University

"Gibbs ends his sometimes sad but utterly beautifully told journey with a message of hope. As the understanding about Alzheimer's disease progresses, more evidence is gained to prevent it. In the wake of a drug that will cure this disease, there is now overwhelming evidence that life style choices (such as exercise, a Mediterranean diet, mentally stimulating activities, social engagement, and good sleep) might markedly slow down its progression. In Gibbs' own words: "I set out to write this book to normalize [that] conversation so that more people can learn about [those] possibilities in time to make a difference. I realize now that some of the lessons I've learned along the way speaks to the fear and dread, as well as the hopes and gifts of life in the moment we have, whatever we face"."

Lancet Neurol 2013; 12: 129–30

A Tattoo on My Brain

A Neurologist's Personal Battle against Alzheimer's Disease

DANIEL GIBBS
Emeritus of Oregon Health and Science University

TERESA H. BARKER
Freelance journalist and author of scientific non-fiction

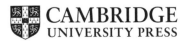

CAMBRIDGE
UNIVERSITY PRESS

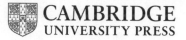
CAMBRIDGE
UNIVERSITY PRESS

Shaftesbury Road, Cambridge CB2 8EA, United Kingdom

One Liberty Plaza, 20th Floor, New York, NY 10006, USA

477 Williamstown Road, Port Melbourne, VIC 3207, Australia

314–321, 3rd Floor, Plot 3, Splendor Forum, Jasola District Centre,
New Delhi – 110025, India

103 Penang Road, #05-06/07, Visioncrest Commercial, Singapore 238467

Cambridge University Press is part of Cambridge University Press & Assessment,
a department of the University of Cambridge.

We share the University's mission to contribute to society through the pursuit of
education, learning and research at the highest international levels of excellence.

www.cambridge.org
Information on this title: www.cambridge.org/9781009325189
DOI: 10.1017/9781009330961

First published 2021
Second edition 2023

Printed in the United Kingdom by TJ Books Limited, Padstow Cornwall

A catalogue record for this publication is available from the British Library.

ISBN 978-1-009-32518-9 Paperback

For all our children and grandchildren, the next generations around the world,

in the hope and expectation that, with our hard work and dedication,

Alzheimer's disease can be beaten

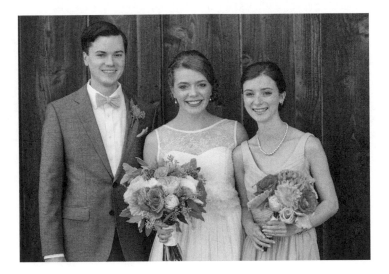

CONTENTS

ACKNOWLEDGMENTS

Dr. Gil Rabinovici at University of California–San Francisco (UCSF) first asked me to write about my experiences with early-stage Alzheimer's disease as seen through the eyes of both patient and neurologist. He has graciously allowed me to reproduce several of his images. He has become a friend and colleague as well as one of my physicians. Other neurologists who have provided medical care, encouragement and/or information for this book include: at Oregon Health & Science University (OHSU), Drs. Joe Quinn, Jeff Kaye, Dennis Bourdette, Marissa Kellogg, Lisa Silbert and Kirsten Wright; at UCSF, Drs. Richard Tsai and Lawren VandeVrede; and, at the Alpert Medical School of Brown University, Dr. Steve Salloway.

This book would not exist without the help of my cowriter, Teresa Barker. Teresa saw promise in my initial linear, and somewhat pedantic, memoir. She reorganized the structure, gave me almost daily writing assignments, and finally produced a much more readable and interesting narrative. Thanks to Lauren Kessler for introducing me to Teresa. We also extend our appreciation to Teresa's family, and to Suzanne Shellenbarger, Wendy Miller and her late husband Gene Cohen, and Stephanie Tade, for their insights and enthusiasm.

Our agent Madeleine Morel believed in this book from the start of my collaboration with Teresa. Thank you, Madeleine, for understanding and supporting my desire to work with an academic publisher. Our editor at Cambridge University Press, Anna Whiting, was so enthusiastic about the book from the start. She and the marketing, editing and design teams at the University Press came through in a really big way to marshal *Tattoo* from manuscript to finished book in what seemed to be lightning speed.

Erin Grace Porozni (www.eringracephotography.com) enthusiastically gave me her permission to use two photographs she took at my daughter Elizabeth's wedding. Dennis Cunningham, one of my favorite Oregon artists, graciously allowed me to reproduce his block print "B is for Beacon."

My daughter Susannah Gibbs, a postdoctoral fellow in public health, was an early reader of the manuscript, and was extraordinarily helpful running down references and helping me understand some statistical concepts. My other daughter, Elizabeth Gibbs, and son, Adam Gibbs, were very supportive and never shy about offering their opinions and feedback. And I am grateful to Elizabeth's husband, Nick Fenster, for his generous help with video elements of the book's online presence.

Finally, I want to thank Lois Seed, my partner in life for fifty-one years, in marriage for forty-eight years, and in this book project for more than two years. It wouldn't have happened without you.

INTRODUCTION

I am a retired neurologist with early-stage Alzheimer's disease. Although I cared for many patients with Alzheimer's disease and other dementias during my career, it never occurred to me that I might one day have it too. I do. So now I'm on the patient's side of the experience, an expert from the inside out on my own early-stage Alzheimer's as it stakes out its slowly growing presence in my brain

The operative phrase here is "slowly growing." Most Alzheimer's patients are diagnosed when symptoms of the disease show up in their behavior or cognitive functioning – they may seem noticeably "off" to those who know them or to themselves. That's typically around the time that the damage to brain cells has become moderate to severe. I found mine much earlier because I went looking for it. It was a fluke, really, that I stumbled across some genetic information that prompted my clinical search. It's easy to say I'm unlucky to have Alzheimer's. But in truth, I'm lucky to have found what I found when I found it. That has meant all the difference, as it has enabled me to access cutting-edge medicine through clinical trials and other progressive treatment options. And I've made some simple lifestyle choices about diet, exercise and social and intellectual activity that evidence-based science has found beneficial for brain health and resilience, including for those with Alzheimer's. Along the way, I've also discovered that nature itself is an impartial guide on this journey. Whether it is in cells viewed through the most sophisticated technology, the earth underfoot on a walk, or the currents that shape a day on the river, the lessons emerge. As a scientist and physician, I want to share this lifeline with others.

It might seem that *early-stage* Alzheimer's disease, with imperceptible or only mild cognitive impairment, has little to teach anyone outside a highly specialized subset of neurologists and research scientists who work with it. I suggest otherwise. In the most universal sense, a diagnosis of Alzheimer's disease is clarifying; it presents the uninvited opportunity to confront your own mortality and get serious about making the most of the time you have. In concrete terms, the sooner you know a disease process has begun, the sooner you can take reasonable steps to stop or slow that process and review your other life priorities. What's really important to accomplish in the time you have left, perhaps checking that bucket list and strengthening connections to friends and relatives. At a societal level, science and statistics show a perfect storm already under way and growing around Alzheimer's: incidence of the disease escalating, a shortage of medical and care specialists, an overwhelming burden on primary care physicians who are underprepared and inadequately trained to provide effective care, and an unimaginable struggle for families and patients themselves. This is no small subset of Americans. Some 5.8 million American are living with Alzheimer's dementia today, a figure projected to reach 14 million by 2050. The world-wide prevalence of Alzheimer's disease and related dementias was estimated to be 35 million in 2010 and expected to rise to 115 million by 2050 [1]. Most dementia patients in high-income countries are diagnosed at the moderate to advanced stage, when noticeable symptoms first prompt medical attention. In limited-resource settings, many people never receive care for dementia or arrive at a hospital or clinic only in the end-stages of their disease.

Dementia is a degenerative disorder of the brain that causes loss of memory and disturbances in thought processing in excess of those of normal aging. These changes in the brain impair a person's ability to perform everyday tasks and activities, and affect their ability to communicate with others – listen and respond – and maintain their part in relationships. Alzheimer's disease accounts for at least 60 percent of cases of dementia, although other causes, including Parkinson's disease, can sometimes be difficult to distinguish from Alzheimer's by symptoms alone and sometimes occur in combination with Alzheimer's in the same person.

A definitive diagnosis of Alzheimer's disease requires evidence of the amyloid plaques (clumps of protein fragments) and neurofibrillary tangles (twisted fibers formed from another kind of protein) in the brain that were discovered by Dr. Alois Alzheimer in 1906. Until relatively recently, this evidence could only be obtained by examining the brain microscopically after death. Now there are biomarker tests that can provide good information about the presence of Alzheimer's pathology during life. These include spinal fluid tests for the amyloid protein found in the plaques and the abnormal tau protein found in neurofibrillary tangles. PET scans of the brain can now show the location of these proteins, and blood tests for both amyloid and tau may be available soon.

Research using these biomarkers has shown that the first abnormality in the brain of a person with Alzheimer's, the formation of plaques, starts to occur up to twenty years before there are any cognitive symptoms – signs of dementia. The tangles and subsequent death of nerve cells that result in brain atrophy start about the time of the first symptoms of cognitive impairment or even a few years before. This realization that abnormalities in the Alzheimer's brain start years before any symptoms occur has led to the idea that effective, disease-modifying treatment would ideally be started in the earliest stages of the disease, perhaps well before there are any symptoms.

Traditionally, Alzheimer's disease has been synonymous with Alzheimer's dementia. A diagnosis of Alzheimer's disease depended on symptoms of dementia being present. Some experts in the field still hold to this strict definition. That's begun to change, however, in the past two decades, since we've learned conclusively that the pathological changes in the brain start ten to twenty years before there is any cognitive impairment. Many experts now hold that we should include in our definition of the disease these pre-symptomatic years when the brain changes are occurring but cognition is still normal, so that interventions to slow that disease process could start sooner. I am one of them.

While experts in my field continue to debate how to define early-stage Alzheimer's in diagnostic terms, we have tests that can spot the disease process under way, affording precious time for those like me, who could be taking steps that evidence-based science suggests can slow the cognitive decline of Alzheimer's disease. I only wish these tests had been available through the many years when the first I saw of Alzheimer's patients was when they were referred to me with cognitive impairment already well advanced.

I have retired from practice, but that just means I've had more time to devote to raising awareness about early-stage Alzheimer's and what we can do about it.

In the fall of 2018, three years after my diagnosis and five years after my retirement, one of my neurologists at the UCSF Memory and Aging Center encouraged me to write a paper directed to neurologists about my experiences as a patient with Alzheimer's disease. In that paper, published in *JAMA Neurology* in spring of 2019, I strongly advocated for early awareness and diagnosis of Alzheimer's [2]. The reasons have only become more compelling with the passage of time:

- New studies continue to advance the scientific understanding of the genetic and other biological and environmental factors that converge to cause Alzheimer's and other forms of dementia. They show a more nuanced view of the disease progression. At the same time, other new studies underscore the protective benefits that diet, physical and mental exercise, social activity, and potentially some medications provide against neurodegenerative decline, including Alzheimer's.

- Innovative genetic technologies are swiftly transforming possibilities, at times so swiftly that they challenge the more deliberate and cautious presentation of medical information customary in generations past. Ancestry trackers like 23&Me and Ancestry.com provide individualized genetic data for customers who want to see theirs. This easy access for consumers can be helpful. But the methods any company uses to harvest the data, the quality of it and how individuals will interpret it and act on it – often without ever consulting their doctor or a genetic counselor – leaves users vulnerable.

- The number of clinical trials for drugs and other therapeutics searching for a way to slow the progress of neurodegenerative disease has increased dramatically, meaning that there are more opportunities for individuals to participate, and more opportunity for doctors to flag relevant clinical trials for a patient's consideration.

We continue to see mounting evidence for gains possible in identifying Alzheimer's at the earliest stages, to slow or even stop cell damage, years before symptoms might predictably emerge. The hope for the future is unfolding on multiple fronts, with progress emerging every day in the urgent quest to bring the best in medical science from bench to bedside.

Meanwhile, media coverage of Alzheimer's and related research are often highly technical, frequently conflicting, and sometimes over-simplified and misleading, creating more confusion than clarity about Alzheimer's disease and what can be done about it. Well before the coronavirus crisis struck, the steady stream of Alzheimer's news had led to a kind of update fatigue for many, especially those keen to see new research findings deliver quick results bedside. All the more so today, slowing the progression of the disease and the move by so many to nursing care facilities are imperative. My hope with this book is to help readers see the mosaic of findings in a more practical and helpful picture. While no single study has cracked the code for an immediate cure, each one contributes to our understanding in ways that eventually will lead to more effective treatment and prevention. In the meantime, we are not helpless, but the fear and stigma of Alzheimer's can make us feel that we are.

Despite the advances that support earlier diagnosis and treatment of Alzheimer's, assumptions of helplessness and despair have dominated the public conversation. The same is often true in the medical community. Urged by colleagues, I began writing this book as an expansion of that *JAMA Neurology* paper published in 2019, to press for change in the medical profession, especially among those physicians on the front lines with patients who might benefit. But there's no reason that, as individuals, we have to wait for institutional change. We can take reasonable, responsible evidence-based steps to help ourselves.

There is so much at stake in any one person's life. Years of cherished shared time with loved ones, as I have enjoyed with my wife, children and grandchildren. Years to enjoy our favorite things, and friends, colleagues and others in so many ways. All of us – those with Alzheimer's or at high risk of it, families, friends and caregivers, researchers and research funders, the healthcare industry and public policy makers – we all stand to gain.

Alzheimer's at any stage is a tough disease, in part because, at any age or stage, just knowing that you're living with it is enough to upend assumptions you may have had about the future. It calls for conversations that may be tough, too, whether that conversation is with your doctor, family, friends or others. Among my patients and others I've known who've received a difficult diagnosis, some choose to bare their innermost feelings, others don't. Everyone has their own coping style. I respect them all. As for me, as odd as it might seem, I'm fascinated by this disease that, for my entire career as a scientist and a neurologist, I could only observe from the outside. Now I've got a front-row seat – or, rather, I'm in the ring with the tiger. Of course I'm disappointed that I have Alzheimer's. But I'm stuck with it. And the habits of a lifetime – to approach a question with a certain kind of detachment and to study, experiment, hypothesize and discover – turn out to be my coping mechanisms. I'm grateful for that now. I hope that this book, informed by that perspective on the science, medicine and everyday life experience of early-stage Alzheimer's, will be of help to others.

Following publication of my essay in *JAMA Neurology*, KATU-TV in Portland featured me in a story about the importance of early diagnosis. I was surprised by the number of people who saw it and commented (https://katu.com/news/local/retired-neurologist-with-alzheimers-shares-importance-of-early-awareness).

Just like that, my diagnosis went from private to public, and my wife Lois and I heard from lots of people – neighbors who hadn't known, or total strangers, many with sad condolences or sympathy. It could be awkward, honestly, since I was for all practical purposes fine – able and active – while many of them had far more difficult things going on in their lives. That is especially true today, as the Covid-19 pandemic has forced us all to confront our mortality, to grieve losses and, for many, to live in dread of an uncertain future.

What we realized in early 2019 was that the conversation about Alzheimer's had long been stuck on fast-forward to the late stage, end-stage loss, the fear and stigma of the disease, not recognizing the years – even decades – of meaningful time that can be maximized with early diagnosis and treatment. I set out to write this book to normalize that conversation so that more people can learn about those possibilities in time to make a difference. I realize now that some of the lessons I've learned along the way speak to the fears and dread, as well as the hopes and gifts of life in the moment we have, whatever we face.

Most narratives about Alzheimer's understandably focus on the emotional impact of the loss or struggle as the disease advances. My purpose is different: to illuminate the potential of a biologically unique and irreplaceable period of time in which we have the opportunity to change the course of Alzheimer's in any one person's life. This is not false hope or Pollyanna thinking. This is evidence-based medical science, partnered with established findings of the benefits that exercise, diet, social activity and cognitive challenge have been shown to have in regard to the progression of Alzheimer's disease. I share my story not as clinical proof, but simply as medical parable and a call to action for anyone who might be open to encouragement. In the context of the times, I hope this message of optimism adds a sense of agency when we may otherwise feel helpless against the disease.

My experience as someone living with early-stage Alzheimer's gives me the insider's vantage point – one that no one would welcome but which I accept and engage in as an opportunity to continue my life's work. My motivation is two-fold: Personally, I want to live fully and savor the time I have with those I love, doing the things I love.

Professionally, as a physician, and earlier as a research scientist, my purpose has always been to help others. This book embodies my determination to continue to work in whatever capacity I can, to do as much as I can for as long as I can, to benefit as many as possible.

The challenge and pleasure of writing this book – living this book – are all the more intensely felt in some ways as holding my own against Alzheimer's and making the most of the time I have. Against any chronic degenerative disease, clinicians measure the success of treatment by its contribution to "a meaningful outcome." For any of us, I believe, that is the universally desired outcome: a life with meaning. That is the story of *A Tattoo on My Brain*.

Chapter-references

1   Prince M, Bryce R, Albanese E, *et al*. The global prevalence of dementia: a systemic review and meta-analysis. *Alzheimer's & Dementia* 2013; 9:63–75; https://doi.org/10.1016/j.jalz.2012.11.007.
2   Gibbs, DM. Early awareness of Alzheimer disease: a neurologist's personal perspective. *JAMA Neurology* 2019; 76:249; https://doi.org/10.1001/jamaneurol.2018.4910.

PROLOGUE

When Auguste D. was about 52, her husband noticed she was acting oddly, misplacing things around the house and suspecting him of having an affair with the next-door neighbor. Her memory rapidly declined over the next year and her paranoia and delusions worsened. The year was 1901, and she was admitted to the Asylum for the Insane and Epileptic in Frankfurt, where she came under the care of Dr. Alois Alzheimer, a young German psychiatrist with an interest in trying to link neuropathological changes in the brain with psychiatric and neurological illnesses. At the time Auguste D. died in 1906, Dr. Alzheimer had moved to another position in Munich, but he was able to obtain her brain for pathological examination. Under the microscope, he saw dark particles between the nerve cells in the outer layers of the brain. He also saw a different type of smaller dark particles within the nerve cells, which were twisted in appearance. These were the plaques and tangles in the brain that we recognize today as the signature of Alzheimer's disease, the neurodegenerative disease named for the doctor who first correlated this specific pathology in the brain with a form of dementia.

Auguste D. died just five years after first seeing Dr. Alzheimer, and probably about eight or nine years after her husband first noticed her unusual behavior. More than a hundred years have passed since Auguste's diagnosis and death, and yet the typical time from diagnosis to death for those with Alzheimer's disease has remained the same, about eight years.

That was the prognosis that I saw play out for most Alzheimer's patients in my twenty-five years as a clinical neurologist. By the time their symptoms brought them to me, the disease had typically progressed beyond anything medicine could do. Today, neuroscience has advanced to the point that we know now that Alzheimer's disease starts in the brain at least ten, possibly twenty, years before any cognitive symptoms are noticed. The question is, with earlier detection of the changes that set the stage for neurodegenerative disease, could we stop those processes before the damage is done, acting to change the course of this disease? Can we use that lead time to buy time against Alzheimer's? I believe the answer is yes. I know because I'm living it.

1 BEACON ROCK

A towering stump of basalt second only to the Rock of Gibraltar, Beacon Rock rises 848 feet from the Washington shore of the Columbia River, about 40 miles east of my home on the Oregon side, up a dead-end street in a woodsy hilltop neighborhood in Portland. The river feels like my second home, carrying years of memories and the promise of more good times spent on the water, first with my kids when they were kids, and now with my grandchildren. This is where they learned some lessons in resourcefulness and practical skills for life and where I learned some of the ropes myself.

Those days are numbered now, though the timeline is imprecise. Ordinarily, this would be maddening for me as a former research scientist and neurologist for whom precision is second nature. But I'm officially retired now, leaving me free to pursue any research I wish, and the whole point of my current project is to exploit this imprecise timeline confronting me and discover how to tweak it in my favor – turn the uncertainty of it to my advantage.

I have early-stage Alzheimer's disease, the beginnings of neurodegenerative processes that will progress over time and someday kill me if something else doesn't get me first. My interest now lies in navigating the progression of this disease in its early stages to find ways to slow it down. I want to buy myself more time on this end of the Alzheimer's continuum. Time with my family and friends. Time to study, read and write, for professional purposes as well as pleasure. Time to enjoy walks in the woods and time on the river. The good news is, I've discovered that all of these pursuits intersect. Each informs the others, advancing some aspect of the larger inquiry around science or life satisfaction, or setting up for the step of insight that will. How that all fits together neurologically – how a brisk walk affects the way your brain functions, for instance – is really pretty amazing in the landscape of the brain. For now, Beacon Rock is a good place to start.

On a clear day, the Portland skyline is dwarfed by nearby Mount Hood, a sleepy volcano, and some sister peaks that thrill hiking enthusiasts. I've never been one of them. But, about five years ago, when I suspected that I had some very early signs of Alzheimer's disease, my thoughts turned to the bucket list of things I wanted to do in my lifetime. Years of volunteer work as a neurologist assisting at the Kilimanjaro Christian Medical Centre (KCMC) in Tanzania had put Mt. Kilimanjaro in my sights.

About that time, on one of my continuing annual volunteer trips to the region, my wife Lois came too, and we took a day hike to Mandara Hut, considered the first full stop for camping and allowing time to acclimatize to the altitude and to the physical exertion required to complete the climb to Kilimanjaro's summit.

One of the unique aspects of working with staff at the hospital in the foothills of Mt. Kilimanjaro is the exposure to patients with high-altitude sickness and other climbing misadventures. Mt. Kilimanjaro is just short of 20,000 feet tall, the tallest mountain in Africa, but climbing it does not require technical climbing skills. It can be done by almost anyone. But it is physically demanding and can be deadly. Each year, about 40,000 climbers attempt to summit, and on average about 6 to 10 of them die trying. About 60 percent of deaths on the mountain are due to high-altitude sickness; 30 percent to medical illnesses such as heart attack, pneumonia or appendicitis; and about 10 percent to trauma from falls or being struck by rocks. In

2013, a famous Irish mountaineer was killed by lightning while climbing the mountain. High-altitude headache occurs in about 80 percent of unacclimatized climbers who have recently reached about 10,000 feet. It can usually be relieved by good hydration, simple analgesics and allowing time for acclimatization. The next step in severity is acute mountain sickness which combines headache with loss of appetite, nausea with vomiting or diarrhea, and sleepiness. The most severe stage is high-altitude cerebral edema. In addition to the severe headache and gastrointestinal symptoms of acute mountain sickness, the climber suffers confusion, loss of coordination, trouble speaking, and lassitude progressing to coma and death if not treated immediately. It is often associated with high-altitude pulmonary edema – the accumulation of fluid in the lungs that causes difficulty breathing. This occurs in about 1 percent of climbers above 15,000 feet. Most people recover fully if immediately transported to a lower elevation, but residual changes in the eye (retinal hemorrhages) and brain (microhemorrhages) may be seen months later [1].

It took us about four hours to climb from the Marangu trailhead to a spot at about 9,000 feet. Even at this relatively low elevation – only about halfway to the top – both of us had mild symptoms of headache and queasiness. The symptoms rapidly improved as we descended the mountain, and once we returned home I was stoked to try again next year – for the summit. Lois thought this was a seriously bad idea, considering my high risk now for potentially lethal neurological complications, such as those from altitude sickness.

Lois wouldn't agree to go with me, so I asked my friend Henry, a seasoned trekker, if he'd join me. Henry suggested I train for it and offered to help me start to get in shape with some local hiking and climbing – perhaps eventually to summit Mount Hood, which he'd done many times. We started with modest day hikes in the Columbia River

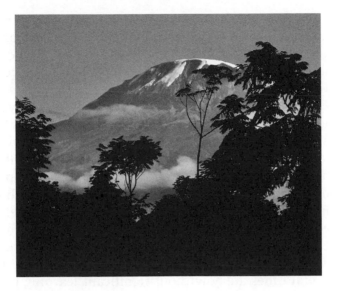

Mt. Kilimanjaro as seen from the KCMC campus where I worked in Tanzania.

Gorge, and by the time I sensibly realized that Lois was right – Mt. Kilimanjaro was out of the question – Henry had introduced me to Beacon Rock.

At a glance, Beacon Rock looks daunting. The south face is. A 400-foot vertical climb reserved for experienced rock climbers only, it requires technical skill and equipment. But the west face, adapted more than a century ago for use by more casual weekend walkers, features wooded trails and an elaborate scaffolding of fifty-four switchbacks, some of them wide footpaths carved into the rock, others spanning wooden bridges (seventeen of them) and walkways, all lined with safety rails. If heights bother you, then it's easy enough to look straight ahead along the broad footpaths and pause to enjoy the scenic distant vistas. It's only scary if you look down the steep rock face.

The views from the riverbank and forest trailhead below and the summit are breathtakingly beautiful. Every step along the way is a walk through woods and rocky terrain that exist in geological time, millions of years in the making and absent any sense of urgency. There's something calming about that for me. A day on the river and the rock quickens the senses, and for me carries years of memories and current good times spent on the water with my family and friends. Once a year now, Henry and I do the mile-plus hike up. At the summit, the bald rock narrows as it juts upward still, and the last 50 feet or so of the engineered path follows concrete steps, a 45-degree Stairmaster climb to the top.

On my most recent hike up Beacon Rock, as I reach the top I feel a little winded, definitely sweaty, but also exhilarated with the pure joy of this incredible workout in my most favorite place. I am participating in a clinical trial of a new smartphone-based cognitive test that can be taken several times a day without significant learning bias – meaning it doesn't get easier with repetition. The goal of the trial is to see whether fluctuations in cognition can be linked to activity level. The cognitive data from the smartphone app is correlated with measures of exercise obtained through a fitness tracker. Lately, although I've started to notice some decline in cognition, more forgetfulness and befuddlement, I still think more clearly during and after exercise. This has been borne out in this study so far. On average, my cognitive assessment score increases 8 percent after aerobic exercise. Today, my fitness tracker says my heart rate is 131, up from a baseline of 64 at the start of the hike. After the 1.75-mile, 57-minute hike from the boat dock to the top of Beacon Rock, elevation gain 850 feet, the cognitive assessment score has increased by 15 percent.

I mention this later to a friend, who laughs at my endless interest in data even on a day when I'm out in this gorgeous natural setting. But for me, this sophisticated tracking program, the real-time feedback and the fact that it's part of a clinical trial only add to my enjoyment of the hike. Like the rock climbers who prefer the hard way up

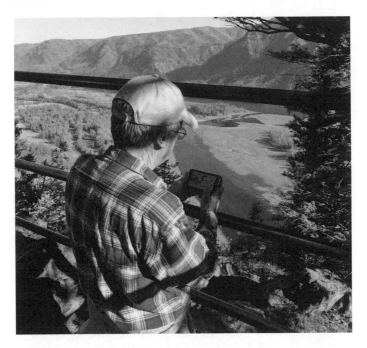

Taking a cognitive test on the summit of Beacon Rock. Photo by my friend John Harland.

the rock face, I take pleasure in the gritty detail of the data. It's an inward-facing vista for me I can appreciate – an encouraging one for now – without taking a thing away from the trail views.

Hikers like us don't run into the rock climbers, whose treacherous ascent up the south face rewards them with a different viewpoint. But any way you look out at the gorge, it's spectacular. I'm just grateful that the easier trail option exists. It's the switchbacks that make the climb possible at all for me, however challenging it is on any given day.

Sometimes the thought of the years ahead with Alzheimer's feels especially daunting, a towering monolith, a sheer rock face. At those times, I think of Beacon Rock, the gift of switchbacks and the power of one step at a time.

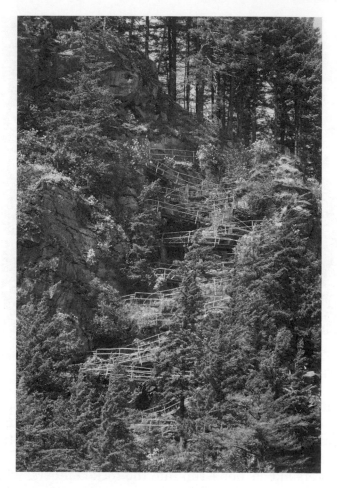

Switchbacks on the face of Beacon Rock.

Chapter-reference

1   Dekker MCJ, Wilson MH, Howlett WP. Mountain
     neurology. *Practical Neurology* 2019; 19:404–411;
     https://doi.org/10.1136/practneurol-2017-001783.

2 FOREWARNED AND FOREARMED

It's not as if I don't know what's in store at the far end of Alzheimer's. For nearly thirty years, most of the Alzheimer's patients I saw in my practice were already in moderate to advanced stages of the disease when their doctors referred them to me.

One patient – I'll call her M. – enters my thoughts now as vividly as the moment she arrived for her appointment. M. was in her eighties, a little unsteady on her feet, so I walked her into my office. Her daughter, with whom she lived, followed closely behind. The daughter had brought her mother to see me because M. had been getting increasingly forgetful, repeating herself all the time. She had been living by herself until recently, but her daughter realized that M. couldn't safely live independently anymore. Her primary care doctor had already ordered a brain MRI scan that showed brain atrophy but no strokes or tumors. As we went through the standard neurological exam, M.'s responses were notable for poor verbal memory – she wasn't able to recall three words I had named five minutes before. She also had some trouble showing me how she would comb her hair or brush her teeth. She had a slightly unsteady gait and on the Mini-Mental Status Exam she scored 12 out of 30. M. had dementia, and clinically it was most consistent with Alzheimer's disease. She didn't seem particularly worried, but her daughter was clearly upset.

Another patient, in her mid-fifties and relatively young on the dementia spectrum, had very early but clear signs of cognitive impairment when she came alone to see me.

When she shared her foremost concerns with me, they were for her family – not for herself. She feared the impact of a diagnosis on them. She didn't want the diagnosis, or her condition, to become the focus of family life, a chronic burdensome concern for those she loved. She wanted to spare them at whatever cost to herself, even if it meant struggling by herself until she couldn't hide her condition any longer.

As a doctor, I hated this disease. It was 1992, and medicine had nothing to offer. Not even hope. Hopelessness was usually already evident by the time patients and their families met with me. As with M., their primary care physicians were at a loss to offer any treatment options, and so I was the next step down a dreaded slippery slope. Many patients already feared the worst, for themselves as well as their families. Neurologists at that time had very limited tools to make even a diagnosis of Alzheimer's before death, much less offer targeted treatment. PET scans were not generally available so we were limited to MRI and CT scans to rule out some of the conditions that mimic aspects of Alzheimer's, like certain brain tumors, strokes and other abnormalities. Much later, spinal fluid exams were developed that could measure levels of amyloid and tau. None of these tests was definitive, and there was always uncertainty whether a given patient truly had Alzheimer's disease or had a different type of dementia – or even a combination of two or more of these. The distinctions matter because any treatment, to be effective, must address the specific biological mechanisms involved in the dementia.

In the last five to ten years of my neurology practice, I started to see a few patients who were still in the mild cognitive impairment stage of dementia. Some of these patients seemed to benefit from available drugs – some of them significantly. But others didn't. All we knew then was that most of these patients would progress to a state of complete loss of memory and total dependence on others for activities of daily living, and death would come in eight to ten years no matter what we did. There was no reliable way to slow down the inexorable march of this disease.

At that time, hope had little of substance to build upon. Scientists were digging, trying to create the foundations for effective clinical treatments that could translate quickly to our patients. But until the necessary early research on Alzheimer's could identify the most promising ground for new studies, there was only the crudest of maps with which to work. Today, those maps are literally high-definition images on scans that take us into the brain and into the Alzheimer's disease process. It is the difference between the GPS in my car and the floppy paper road maps we once relied upon. These advances, and extensive research showing that lifestyle changes can slow the progression of Alzheimer's, have redefined the territory for treatment and the meaning of hope. Yet, early diagnosis remains an academic discussion while the diagnosis of Alzheimer's continues to come typically when the symptoms – and the damage – are well along, well into the moderate or late stage of the disease. The result can be too little too late to make a meaningful difference, leaving patients and their families desperate as they consider the future.

I correspond from time to time with Greg O'Brien, a journalist, who wrote *On Pluto: Inside the Mind of Alzheimer's* in 2014 about his ongoing experiences with moderately severe Alzheimer's. The Alzheimer's Association originally put us in touch. We soon became friends and, for several years, enjoyed comparing notes by email and phone calls. He is a couple of years ahead of me in his journey, so I learned a lot from him about what to expect. I was the neurologist, but he was living the disease and had the personal experience that I lacked. Both of Greg's parents had died with Alzheimer's, and, in his early fifties, he too started having signs of cognitive impairment. The early onset of his Alzheimer's was apparently due to a severe head injury suffered in a bike accident, combined with his genetic predisposition. Through his increasingly difficult struggle with the disease, Greg continued to be an advocate for greater public awareness of Alzheimer's disease. We've stayed in touch through occasional emails, although, as his condition has worsened, the length of time between responses has grown. More recently, when I don't hear back from him for a while, I check the obituaries. I'm relieved when I don't find him there, and when I do eventually hear back, however much his condition has deteriorated, he is still in the fight. In a recent email, he was blunt and unsentimental about the ravages of the disease at this late stage, describing "symptoms that include horrific short-term memory loss, failure to recognize familiar people, loss of judgment and filter, out-of-control rage, seeing things that aren't there, and others." He emphasized that his fight now isn't to buy himself more time, but to rally resources to help others sooner.

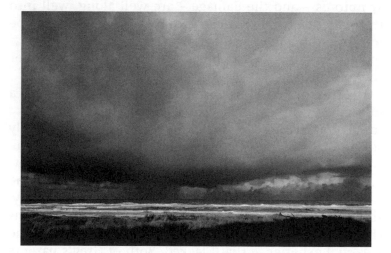

Approaching storm on the Oregon coast.

"I have no interest in prolonging this," he wrote of his own circumstances, "and would prefer that researchers focus their limited resources on pre-symptomatic individuals."[1]

And who might that be? Absent the symptoms, how can you tell? What does Alzheimer's look like when you can't yet see it in someone's behavior? What does it look like in the years before it shows itself?

---

[1] I have directly quoted Greg O'Brien from his personal emails to me with his explicit permission.

3 THE SMELL OF BAKING BREAD

It was a summer day in 2006 when I first noticed that there might be a problem with my ability to smell. Lois and I were walking the dog when we passed some beautiful roses. I leaned over to smell them, but there was hardly any smell. I said to Lois that as beautiful as these roses were, they didn't seem to have much of a scent. Some varieties of roses are like that. Then Lois stepped over, took a sniff and had no trouble getting the usual olfactory treat. The problem wasn't the roses. I didn't think much about it until a year later when I suddenly began experiencing intrusive smells that didn't seem to have any origin in the real world. The smell was always the same: like a mixture of baking bread and perfume. It would occur seemingly out of nowhere and last from a few minutes up to an hour.

These false odors are called *phantosmias* – a kind of olfactory hallucination. In the medical literature, phantosmias are usually associated with decreased ability to smell. It's as though the brain is inventing a smell to replace the one it can no longer detect. Phantosmias are more common in those who have had head injuries, and they are twice as common in people in poor health compared to those in good health [1].

In addition to my fading ability to smell (*hyposmia*) and the false odors characteristic of phantosmia, I would have distortions of true odors, or *dysosmia*. This was particularly noticeable with very strong, usually noxious odors like those of gasoline, exhaust fumes or a skunk's spray. One weekend on a drive with Lois and some friends, the others in the car remarked on a very strong gasoline smell apparently coming from the car in front of us. I could smell something, but it was nothing like the smell of gasoline, and the odor that I alone smelled persisted for another five or ten minutes, long after the others had stopped smelling anything. None of this struck us as anything but an occasional oddity for the next few years, certainly not a medical concern.

The most common causes of loss or distortion of smell include normal aging, smoking, nasal polyps, allergies, and upper respiratory tract infections including the common cold. Less common causes are head trauma, certain toxic chemicals, some medications, cocaine abuse, tumors impinging on olfactory structures, and radiation for head and neck cancers. Neurological disorders such as Parkinson's and Alzheimer's disease are frequently associated with impaired smell.[1] Leprosy is rarely seen in the US, Canada, the UK and Europe, but it is still relatively common in India, Indonesia, Brazil and parts of Africa,[2] and the bacillus that causes leprosy has a high affinity for the olfactory nerve, so virtually all patients with the disease have significant loss of smell [4]. Nearly all people with COVID-19 have some loss of the ability to smell, often as the first symptom [5].

I'd had no head injuries, I was in good health, I didn't smoke or use cocaine, and my only exposures to chemicals that can affect olfaction were the formaldehyde fumes in

---

[1] The best book I have found on olfactory disturbances from a neurological point of view is *Smell and Taste Disorders*, by CH Hawkes and RL Doty [2]. Chapter 5 covers general disorders of olfaction, and chapter 7 discusses the neurodegenerative diseases including Alzheimer's. The previous edition was titled *The Neurology of Olfaction*.

[2] There are approximately 208,000 yearly new leprosy cases worldwide. The US has only 150 to 250 new cases of leprosy each year. While many of these are thought to be acquired while living or working abroad, in certain parts of the southern US, the majority of cases are caused by transmission of the leprosy bacillus from armadillos to humans [3].

the medical school anatomy lab forty years ago, an unlikely culprit this long after the fact. And although I had seen patients with leprosy in my work at the hospital in Tanzania, they had almost all been treated and were no longer contagious. My risk of getting leprosy was minimal.

I mentioned the smell issues during an annual check-up with my primary care doctor mostly as a curiosity. My doctor was more concerned about it than I was, and insisted on ordering a brain MRI scan. I thought she was overreacting. After all, I'm the neurologist. She's the internist. My mind was fine. I didn't really expect there'd be anything on an MRI scan, but I agreed to schedule one, unconcerned.

Glancing out the window of my doctor's second-floor office, the only thing on my mind was where to pick up a fresh cup of coffee on my stroll back to my car. The view looked out into the treetops of the park-like downtown college campus nearby and the surrounding neighborhood of tree-lined streets, sidewalk cafes and trendy boutiques. The biggest decision in the moment: Starbucks, Peet's or one of the many indie coffee kiosks along the way. They were all my favorites, one of the perks of this lively, eclectic urban neighborhood. Block after block of shaggy shrubs, towering oaks and evergreens, mossy fences and old houses gave the place a homey feel, just as it had thirty-plus years before, when a neurology residency at a major medical center here prompted our move from San Diego.

In San Diego at UCSD for the previous six years, and in Atlanta for medical school the six years before that, I'd been either a medical student, medical intern or research scientist, and Lois a librarian finishing graduate school then working in the public library systems in both cities. We were frugal, and we'd always found the houses "with character," the Craftsman fixer-uppers back when they were just old houses and not yet trendy vintage. When I was offered the position in Portland in the spring of 1986, it seemed crazy to pick up and move here on short notice, but we did it. The sunny spring day we flew up to go house-hunting, we fell in love with the neighborhood, and this old house stood out all the more because it *wasn't* a fixer-upper. It was move-in ready for this frazzled young couple with a 3-year-old, a new baby and a wild-eyed dog in tow. Lois was especially pleased and relieved. The fact that I was starting a neurology residency guaranteed long hours at the hospital for me, and even more for Lois at the helm of home and family, managing all things great and small.

We loved our first summer, all bright skies and sunshine, drives to the coast or time on the river or in the woods. Once the season gave way to the endless rains, we doubted we'd stay once I'd completed the program. Then life happened – our third child was born, and our first two were making friends and putting down their own young roots in the neighborhood and the town. Soon we were,

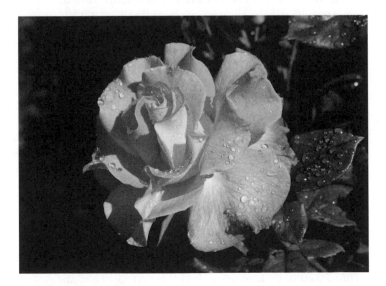

Rose at the International Rose Test Garden in Portland, Oregon.

too. I discovered in the process of completing my residency that I loved working directly with patients, so when the time came and I had the choice to return to research science or continue as a doctor, I chose doctoring and we chose to stay.

As a purely practical matter of my own health care, this meant that through the years, in routine visits with my internist, a friend since residency days, I was a collegial partner in the conversation about clinical details. As it happened, none of my details was ever very interesting. I had always been unremarkable in that sense – the best kind of boring. That was about to change.

Chapter-references

1   Bainbridge KE, Byrd-Clark D, Leopold D. Factors associated with phantom odor perception among US adults. *JAMA Otolaryngology – Head & Neck Surgery* 2018; 144:807–814 (public access version available at www.ncbi.nlm.nih.gov/pmc/articles/PMC6233628).

2   Hawkes CH, Doty RL. *Smell and Taste Disorders.* Cambridge University Press, 2018.

3   Truman RW, Singh P, Sharma R., *et al.* Probable zoonotic leprosy in the southern United States. *New England Journal of Medicine* 2011; 364:1626–1633; www.nejm.org/doi/full/10.1056/NEJMoa1010536 (public access version available at www.ncbi.nlm.nih .gov/pmc/articles/PMC3138484).

4   Mishra A, Saito K, Barbash SE, Mishra N, Doty RL. Olfactory dysfunction in leprosy. *Laryngoscope* 2006; 116:413–416; https://doi.org/10.1097/01.MLG .0000195001.03483.F2.

5   Hawkes CH. Smell, taste and Covid-19: testing is essential [published online ahead of print, 2020 Dec 19]. *QJM* 2020;hcaa326; doi: 10.1093/qjmed/hcaa326.

4 SNEAK PREVIEW

In my neurology practice, when patients had scans or other tests done, we always made an appointment to go over the results together within a few days or a week. The point was that it was something you did together: we looked at the images together, discussed what we saw, talked through their questions, concerns, fears, and talked about next steps. That's the way it's supposed to work.

Since I could access the digital files of my scans myself as a physician, I thought I'd just take a quick look to confirm that this was a non-issue. Save my doctor and myself the trouble of a follow-up appointment. As I pulled up the scan, I wasn't expecting to see anything, so I was startled to see a significant something. I leaned closer and stared at the image on the screen. There was a really big tumor there, a surprisingly *large* tumor – a mass the size of a ping-pong ball. The tumor was arising from my pituitary gland, a bean-size, hormone-producing gland near the base of the brain that controls the activity of most of the other hormone-producing glands in the body, which in turn regulate or influence basically everything else.

Neurology is the branch of medicine that deals with a diverse array of diseases and injuries of the brain, spinal cord, peripheral nerves and muscles. My specialty, building from my early career as a research scientist in neuro-endocrinology and the neurochemistry of stress, meant that I saw patients representing a wide range of mostly chronic neurological conditions, including migraine, multiple sclerosis, peripheral nerve problems, Parkinson's disease and some forms of dementia.

Though I rarely saw patients with pituitary tumors, I knew the tumors are ordinarily benign. But the startling size of this one overwhelmed any rational thoughts I might have had in that moment. What registered was simple shock and pure panic. *I've got cancer in my brain.*

"Oh shit," I declared. "I am so screwed." I thought I was about to die.

I quickly shared the scan with one of my partners in the practice, a neurooncologist who sees tumors all the time. She confirmed that it was a pituitary tumor, likely benign – troublesome, but not malignant. In my case, the tumor was large enough to press against my optic nerve, but fortunately there was no significant effect on

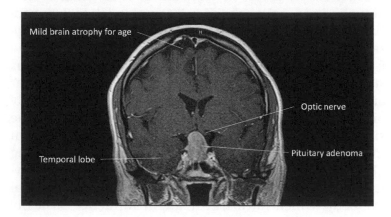

This is an MRI of my brain in 2007. (Age 56.) The view is like a vertical slice through the brain about halfway back. The whitish pituitary tumor can be seen in the middle, pushing up into the optic nerves and outward toward – but not into – the temporal lobes of the brain, home to important memory centers as well as some of the olfactory centers. The radiologist also commented that there was "slightly more brain atrophy than would be expected for this age," an observation that, unrelated to the tumor or any other symptoms, seemed nothing more than an anomaly but may have been a harbinger of things to come.

my vision, at least not yet. My doctor concurred with the diagnosis, and my panic subsided. Everyone agreed that, due to the size of the mass, it should come out, so all I had left to worry about was the nuisance of having to have the surgery, which is pretty unpleasant, but nothing to complain about, given what it could have been. I chose a surgical team at UC San Francisco that specialized in such tumors.

I wasn't particularly anxious about the surgery. I knew it was safe, with a minuscule fatality rate and few complications if done by an experienced surgeon – and mine was well known and respected for his prowess with pituitary tumors. Any potential trauma to the brain itself is much reduced by newer endoscopic surgery techniques that no longer even require entering the brain through the skull – the classic craniotomy procedure in which a portion of the skull is removed to expose the brain. Endoscopic surgery allows the surgeon to access the brain using long thin tubes inserted through the nose and sinus underlying the pituitary gland. I can't say I was disappointed to forgo a craniotomy, but I'd observed many before when my patients needed surgery, and I can't say I would have been disappointed to observe my own.

Early in my training to become a neurologist, when one of my patients had to undergo brain surgery, I watched the operation whenever possible. In those days, brain surgery always started the same way, and the technique and its direct reveal of the brain is still the optimal approach in many cases. First, the neurosurgeon completes a craniotomy to remove a piece of the skull. They then peel back the rough outermost protective layer, the *dura mater*, and the glistening brain is revealed. It has a creamy color, like Edam cheese, with red accents from the blood vessels coursing through and around it. Surprisingly, the brain has no pain sensors, so after the removal of skull and dura, the patient can be awakened from anesthesia and the brain itself can be painlessly manipulated or electrically stimulated, as is sometimes necessary in certain operations for epilepsy or tremor. The patient can report back what they are experiencing during the stimulation. No matter how many of these operations I observed, I was never less awed by one, and by our ability to witness the living brain, so powerful and yet exposed and so vulnerable. As a brain scientist, no doubt I would have found my own surgery interesting to watch. But to witness my own brain now, if only through scans and data, was enough.

With brain cancer off the table now and the tumor no longer appearing to present a serious threat, the rush of relief swept away my concerns and left me with only my usual scientific curiosity. After all, this big pituitary tumor

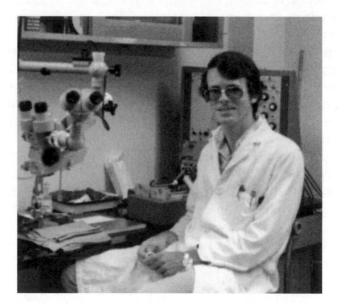

In the lab as a graduate student in 1976 working on my Ph.D. research. Photo by Lois Seed.

was actually quite interesting, and I had a front-row seat in this surgical theatre.[1]

Chapter-reference

1   Gibbs DM, Neill JD. Dopamine levels in hypophysial stalk blood in the rat are sufficient to inhibit prolactin secretion in vivo. *Endocrinology* 1978; 102:1895–1900; http://doi.org/10.1210/endo-102-6-1895.

[1]   There was a huge irony here. As a graduate student, my doctoral dissertation research had involved collecting the pituitary portal blood in rats, the blood that carries releasing factors from the hypothalamus to the pituitary gland. I was able to show that the neurotransmitter dopamine released by the hypothalamus was a physiologically important inhibitor of prolactin secretion from the pituitary. This settled a somewhat contentious debate in the field about whether dopamine played any significant role in prolactin regulation. The paper I wrote with my mentor describing this finding turned out to be the most cited paper of my career. Now, forty years later, all those rats that lost their pituitary glands to benefit my research were getting their revenge [1]!

5 A STUBBORN PUZZLE

A leak in your roof can travel a circuitous route through rafters and joints before it surfaces three rooms away as a creeping stain on the ceiling over your sofa. Symptoms of illness or injury are like the stain, the observable thing that gets your attention and prompts you to investigate further.

Working backward from a symptom to find the cause is the perpetual puzzle of science and medicine. It is particularly so in neurology, with the interconnected complexities of the brain itself, the vast domain of the nervous system, and the mix of hormones and other fluctuating neurochemistry. In any case, the sooner you can track an observable symptom successfully to the source, the sooner you can identify the most effective treatment options.

As our attention turned to this benign tumor and the need to remove it to avoid problems it posed for my optic nerve, I wondered hopefully if it might be the culprit behind my mysterious loss of smell and the strange episodes of imagined smells. If so, puzzle solved. And removal of the tumor would effectively return my sense of smell. My neurosurgeon, who had removed several thousands of these tumors, was quick to quash this theory. He had never seen a pituitary tumor, even the huge ones, cause loss of smell.

I didn't really believe the neurosurgeon. I was almost sure that my sense of smell would begin to come back after the tumor was gone, so I started tracking it with the University of Pennsylvania Smell Identification Test

(UPSIT).[1] Instead of improving after removal of the pituitary tumor, my ability to smell continued to worsen and was completely gone within a few years. The phantosmias, the illusory odors that seemed to come out of nowhere, initially were quite frequent, occurring several times per week. But over the years they became less frequent, occurring just two or three times per year and then disappearing altogether at age 66.

Lois keeps a jigsaw puzzle going almost all the time on the table in our living room, typically the daunting kind with a few thousand pieces that require painstaking sorting and experimenting to assemble. This smell thing had

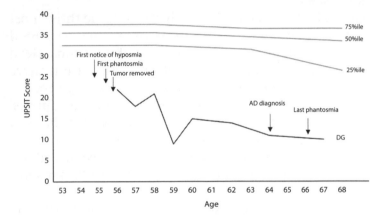

Graph of my scores on the University of Pennsylvania Smell Identification Test (UPSIT) from age 56 to age 67. An average healthy test-taker (50th percentile) will score about 35. A score below 20 indicates severe hyposmia or anosmia. AD, Alzheimer's disease; DG, Daniel Gibbs.

---

[1]   The UPSIT was developed by Dr. Richard L. Doty at the University of Pennsylvania and is one of the most common smell tests used in the US. There are forty scratch-and-sniff cards, each with four choices to choose from. The subject must pick one of the choices, even if she smells nothing. A perfect score is 40. Someone who has absolutely no sense of smell and has to guess randomly will get about ten right. Scores below 20 suggest severe impairment of smell [1].

become my 1,000-piece Escher puzzle. If the pituitary mass was not the cause, then what was? I sorted and re-sorted the puzzle pieces, researching olfactory symptoms and loss in stolen time between my full clinical day, hospital rounds and tucking the kids in at bedtime. These are usually dealt with by ear, nose and throat specialists, the ENTs, and there had been little if any teaching about olfactory disorders in my neurology training. Online research wasn't yet as accessible as it is now, so at times I printed out journal articles at work and lugged them home for my own bedtime reading. *The Neurology of Olfaction* by Christopher H. Hawkes and Richard L. Doty topped my side-table reading stack.

From all of this, I could quickly rule out the three most common causes of olfactory impairment: age over 65 (I was just 56), smoking and chronic nasal infections. Head injuries were a less common but possible cause if there was damage to the olfactory nerves or olfactory processing centers in the brain, but I'd had no head injuries. Next on the list of possibilities, certain diseases that can cause damage to the olfactory bulb, piriform cortex and other smell-processing areas of the brain. I wondered if it could be a neurodegenerative disorder like Parkinson's disease (PD).

As a neurologist, I was well aware of the association between Parkinson's and olfactory disturbances. At least 80 percent of patients with Parkinson's disease have some degree of olfactory impairment, and these changes in the ability to smell can begin ten or more years before any of the other symptoms, such as tremor or trouble walking, occur. The hallucination-like phantosmias have also been reported in Parkinson's patients [2]. At that time, however, there wasn't a widely recognized association between olfactory disturbances and the kinds of neurological conditions that presented in the population of my patients. Most of the Alzheimer's patients I saw in my practice were already in moderate to advanced stages of the disease by the time their doctors referred them to me, and no one mentioned trouble with smelling. Of course, I didn't know to ask.

My olfactory symptoms had been a quirky little medical mystery but not a serious concern of mine before. When removal of the tumor changed nothing about these symptoms, as my neurosurgeon had predicted, I began to stew about the known association with Parkinson's. Although I had absolutely no symptoms suggestive of PD, now I wondered if my loss of smell could be a harbinger of things to come.

Soon enough though, my abstract what-if worry about Parkinson's was eclipsed by my work with patients, expanding administrative and faculty roles at the university medical school, volunteer commitments at home and abroad, and immersion in my own family life. This now included a full family itinerary of sports, Scouts, music, drama, homework, school volunteering, summer camp,

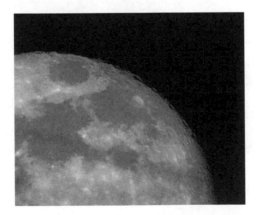

This photo of the supermoon was taken on April 8, 2020 at the moon's perigee, its closest distance to the earth. The full moon appears larger and sharper than usual. The particular pattern of light and shadows later struck me as reminiscent of the skull.

canoe and other field trips, and all the duties and delights of being parents of three growing kids. Years passed. Five years, to be exact. If I felt the clock ticking, it was the same one everyone feels when the passage of time occasionally registers with a sudden awareness. Births, deaths, milestone moments, Kodak moments or sometimes just a glance at the mirror and the surprising sight of an older self peering back.

Chapter-references

1   Doty RL. Olfactory dysfunction and its measurement in the clinic. *World Journal of Otorhinolaryngology – Head and Neck Surgery* 2015; 1:28–33; https://doi.org/10.1016/j.wjorl.2015.09.007 (open access).
2   Landis BN, Burkhard PR. Phantosmias and Parkinson disease. *Archives of Neurology* 2008; 65:1237–1239; https://doi.org/10.1001/archneur.65.9.1237.

6 THE LOCKED BOX AND THE FAMILY TREE

Lois had retired professionally from her career as a librarian when we moved to Portland, but her tenacious appetite for digging and discovery found fertile soil in family life. She became an ardent genealogist – she loves puzzles and loves that genealogy is all about solving puzzles and mysteries. She is as happy digging online as she is digging in the garden – which is to say, very happy. This always led to interesting choices for our rare downtime, and I was a grateful beneficiary of her book and TV viewing recommendations. In 2012, we had become fans of the PBS series *Finding Your Roots* with Henry Louis Gates, Jr., a show that used a combination of traditional genealogical research and DNA testing to trace the family histories of famous people. Around this time, she had been stumped in her efforts to clarify some of the obscure branches of our respective family trees. She suggested that we get our DNA tested by one of the popular ancestry-search companies to see whether that would help.

We had no real thought about what we might discover – perhaps distant family unbeknownst to us, or a past generation's link to a place or way of life new to us. We'd heard interesting tales from friends, as well as in the media, and we thought we might get lucky. Lois was intent on finding those missing pieces of the family picture. Accustomed to road trips and day hikes, now we felt like armchair time travelers as we sent off our saliva swabs for DNA analysis that might find a match from the past.

When our reports arrived online a few weeks later, in addition to a list of potential DNA relatives, there was also access to a list of possible health risks that could be associated with our genes. On the report, there was an icon for a locked box containing results for two genes that were risk factors for neurological diseases. One of these was the LRRK-2 gene. A mutation in this gene is the most common cause of hereditary Parkinson's disease. The other neurological gene test was for apolipoprotein E 4 (APOE-4), the most significant risk factor, other than old age, for late-onset Alzheimer's. To unlock these results, one had to acknowledge that genetic counseling was recommended to interpret the results. Of course I knew that. I checked the box.

At that time, I had not even the slightest hint of Parkinson's symptoms, and I'd almost forgotten that I'd been preoccupied with concern about it some years back. My sense of smell had never returned, but, absent any symptoms of Parkinson's, the active worry had subsided. However, my research into the persistent olfactory issue had brought the LRRK-2 PD gene to my attention, and this snagged it again, if only with mild curiosity. It was a huge relief to open that locked-box folder and see that I did not have the Parkinson's gene.

What I wasn't prepared for was what the test showed I did have. Like the day I pulled up my brain scan and saw that unexpected pituitary tumor, I could hardly believe what I saw on the screen now. I was shocked to discover that I had two copies of the APOE-4 gene, putting me at significant risk of developing Alzheimer's. Both of my parents had died relatively early from cancer, my father at age 60 and my mother at 75, and I'd never seen anything in their behavior that suggested dementia or diminished mental capacity at all. I'd certainly never suspected that either of them carried the genes for Alzheimer's. It hadn't occurred to me that they had died before the age they might have developed symptoms of the disease.

Alzheimer's is just one of many types of dementia, a broadly defined degenerative disorder of the brain that causes loss of memory and thinking in excess of that of normal aging, and results in impairment of a person's ability to perform everyday activities, including work. What we define as Alzheimer's disease accounts for at least 60 percent of cases of dementia, although other causes including vascular dementia, Parkinson's disease, dementia with Lewy bodies, and frontotemporal dementia can sometimes be difficult to distinguish from Alzheimer's by symptoms alone, and in fact can occur in combination with Alzheimer's in the same person. There are many genetic mutations that can increase the risk of getting Alzheimer's, but, so far, the most significant of these for both late-onset and even early-onset Alzheimer's is APOE-4.

It's not as if the APOE gene is designed for destructive purposes; it's not. The APOE gene is the DNA blueprint for a specific lipoprotein, a protein that is involved in the transport for certain lipids in the blood. It comes in three variants, or alleles: APOE-2, APOE-3 and APOE-4. For reasons that are still not entirely clear, this gene for a protein involved in cholesterol transport also affects risk for acquiring Alzheimer's disease. It seems that there is an effect on production of the protein beta-amyloid in the brain, but the mechanism of APOE-4 risk is probably more complicated. We just don't know yet what that is.

Everyone receives one of these alleles from each parent, so, depending on which ones each of your parents gives you, you might have two copies of APOE-2, APOE-3 or APOE-4, or one copy of APOE-2 and one copy of APOE-3, etc. There are six possible combinations. APOE-3 is the most common allele, APOE-2 is least common, and APOE-4 is intermediate. The risk of developing Alzheimer's disease is modestly increased with one copy of APOE-4 and markedly increased with two copies. APOE-3 is considered to provide standard risk, and there is some suggestion that people with APOE-2 have a decreased risk of developing Alzheimer's.

It's important to keep in mind that the APOE-4 allele is a *risk factor* for Alzheimer's, not a determinant. Many people with one copy of APOE-4 will never get Alzheimer's, and even some with two copies will escape the disease. More specifically, the APOE-4-related risk for developing Alzheimer's is this: If you have one copy of APOE-4, your risk for Alzheimer's disease increases about three-fold. If you have two copies, the risk increases about twelve-fold or even higher according to one recent study.[1] Having two copies of APOE-4 also appears to advance the onset of Alzheimer's by about ten years, so someone with two copies of APOE-4 who is going to develop Alzheimer's would be more likely to be diagnosed with late-onset Alzheimer's in his or her early seventies, instead of a typical diagnosis at about age 80. If my DNA results were accurate and I had two copies of the APOE-4 gene, it meant I had about a 50 percent chance of having an Alzheimer's diagnosis by age 70.[2]

---

[1]   In this very detailed study comparing APOE status with autopsy confirmation of Alzheimer's or no Alzheimer's, the risk of getting Alzheimer's disease in those with two copies of APOE-4 was about thirty times higher than in those with two copies of APOE-3 (odds ratio 31.22). Interestingly, the much less common APOE-2 allele appears to be protective. People with two copies of APOE-2 had an odds ratio of 0.13 compared to those with two copies of APOE-3, and an odds ratio of 0.001 compared to two copies of APOE-4: they were 1,000 times less likely to get Alzheimer's [1].

[2]   There is an aspect of the APOE-4 gene that is controversial, but that I find to be fascinating. A number of studies around the end of the 1990s and beginning of the 2000s suggested that young adults who carried the APOE-4 gene performed better on some cognitive tests and/ or were more likely to pursue higher education than their non-APOE-4-carrying peers [2]. One study suggested that this effect was due to a higher neural processing speed in those with APOE-4 [3]. This benefit is

I am not a genetic counselor, but, as a scientist and physician, I'm accustomed to looking at risk factors objectively. They're an important part of weighing the risks and benefits of medications and treatment plans for patients. So now it was my turn on the receiving end of this DNA analysis and the statistical bottom line for my Alzheimer's risk. Once my initial shock at the APOE-4 finding registered, my mind fixed on the data and moved to the bottom line. Yes, someone with the APOE-4 allele is at increased risk, especially if they have two copies. My chances of getting Alzheimer's by age 80 were very high. But some APOE-4 carriers *never get the disease.* This, too, is true. Could I be one of them? Maybe. Maybe not. At the moment, it was impossible to know. Most relevant for me at that time was the objective fact that, although I had two copies of the APOE-4 alleles and thus the elevated risk, I had no signs of cognitive impairment.

There are other risk factors for Alzheimer's, but, knowing that a family history of the disease is a significant one, I started digging, or as one of our kids called our genealogical hunts through overgrown old family cemeteries in Western Pennsylvania, "looking for dead ancestors." A hereditary risk was not obvious in my immediate family, but it didn't take much digging for me to find hints of dementia in previous generations. Tracing a family history of

lost by the mid-fifties, and, after that, the risk for Alzheimer's disease kicks in and cognition worsens [4]. This effect is held out as an example of antagonistic pleiotropy – a gene that is beneficial early in life and harmful later in life. I don't know if this is true, and there is heated debate about it in the field [5], but it resonates with me. I was really smart as a teen and young adult, but I was smart in a lazy kind of way. I just seemed able to think things through faster than my peers, so I could wait to the last minute to do my homework, much to the annoyance of my friends. I remained pretty smart into my sixties when subtle memory issues began, but by then, as we will see, the neuropathological abnormalities of Alzheimer's disease had probably been present in my brain for at least ten years.

diagnosed Alzheimer's disease is not easy. Until the 1970s, Alzheimer's disease was by definition restricted to dementia that occurred before age 65 and had the characteristic amyloid plaques and neurofibrillary tangles when the brain was examined after death. Dementia that began after age 65 was called senile dementia, and it was considered to be a consequence of normal aging, even if a later autopsy showed that the characteristic plaques and tangles were present in the brain.

As Lois combed through new information for leads and whatever details the vestiges of family stories might provide, I scoured the family lore and reexamined old source material with new purpose. Eventually, more clues, patterns and links began to emerge.

My parents' parents, their siblings and extended families presented a mixed legacy of dementia or possible dementia at older ages. Some showed no sign of it at all,

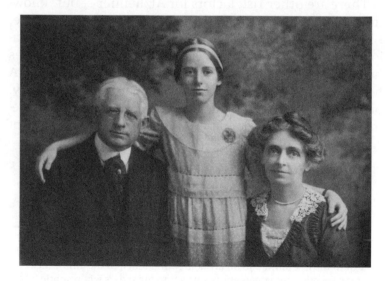

My mother, Elizabeth, center, with my grandparents Daniel and May Martin in about 1920. May probably had dementia in the last few years of her life.

well into older age. Some had died as the result of health complications that might or might not have been related to Alzheimer's. My grandfather Daniel, my mother's father, reportedly had died of a cerebral hemorrhage at age 60 when my mother was just 15 years old. I wonder if he might have had cerebral amyloid angiopathy, a cause of bleeding into the brain that is associated with Alzheimer's disease. Of course, there were no CT scans at the time, and no autopsy was performed. There is some suggestion of odd behavior in his last few years that may have resulted in the loss of his position as pastor of his church in Cynwyd, Pennsylvania, but there was no mention of dementia – or senility as it was called at that time – in the family lore. My mother's mother, my grandmother May, lived to age 78, and, in retrospect, she almost certainly had dementia at the time of her death. There are stories of her wandering in the neighborhood in her night clothes.

My father's parents and grandparents presented a mixed legacy of dementia. His mother, Anna Louise Bosbyshell, died of a stroke at age 81, and there was no obvious sign of dementia. However, her brother, Fred, sister Elsie, and niece all had dementia. My great-uncle Fred had been an eccentric, good-hearted, larger-than-life presence in my life as a kid, and suddenly his final years with Alzheimer's in his mid-eighties took on new meaning. My paternal grandfather, Amelius Marion Gibbs, came to Los Angeles from a farm near Canton, Ohio, in 1899 when he was 22. One of eight siblings, Marion hated life on the farm and left for a job at a bank, working his way up from the bottom to near the top of a Los Angeles bank before dying of a heart attack at age 76. His was a cognitively demanding career and he never showed any evidence of dementia.

Like Lois, I found the genealogy and emerging family story fascinating. Lois had no family history of genetic concerns. But the pieces coming into view for me were

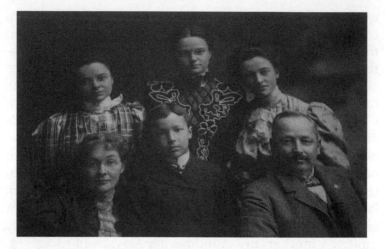

The Bosbyshell family. My paternal grandmother, Anna Louise, is on the right at the back. Her sister Elsie, on the left at the back, and her brother Fred – my great-uncle, whom we all fondly called Uncle Fred – in the center, both had dementia, probably due to Alzheimer's disease.

worrisome. First one, then another. As I connected the dots, the familial constellation of dementia emerged like the outline of some ominous beast against the night sky.

Chapter-references

1 Reiman EM, Arboleda-Velasquez JF, Quiroz YT, *et al.* Exceptionally low likelihood of Alzheimer's dementia in APOE2 homozygotes from a 5,000-person neuropathological study. *Nature Communications* 2020; 11:667; https://doi.org/10.1038/s41467-019-14279-8.
2 Hubacek JA, Pitha J, Škodová Z, *et al.* A possible role of apolipoprotein E polymorphism in predisposition to higher education. *Neuropsychobiology* 2001; 43:200–203; https://doi.org/10.1159/000054890.
3 Rusted JM, Evans SL, King SL, *et al.* APOE 4 polymorphism in young adults is associated with improved attention and indexed by distinct neural

signatures. *NeuroImage* 2013; 65: 364–373; https://doi
.org/10.1016/j.neuroimage.2012.10.010.
4   Jochemsen HM, Muller M, van der Graaf Y, *et al.*
APOE 4 differentially influences change in memory
performance depending on age. The SMART-MR study.
Neurobiology of Aging 2012; 33:832.e15–22 (open access).
5   Ihle A, Bunce D, and Kliegel M. APOE 4 and cognitive
function in early life: a meta-analysis. *Neuropsychology*
2012; 26:267–277; https://doi.org/10.1037/a0026769.

7 THE MEASURE OF MEMORY

Dead reckoning, one of the oldest and most basic methods of navigation, was for centuries an essential piece of the mariner's skill set, and it was still required to captain a charter sailing boat in the late 1990s, when the idea of a late summer week on the water off the San Juan Islands first captured my imagination. The islands, hundreds of them, some inhabited and others no bigger than a pickup truck, form an archipelago off the northernmost coast of Washington and British Columbia. On the water, you share the Salish Sea living room with the likes of baleen whales and orcas, sea lions and otters. The sky is just as lively by day, with the sea birds monitoring the waters for their next meal, and at night – the silent, spectacular sea of twinkling stars.

I learned to sail when I was a kid, growing up near the water in Southern California, where skiffs were common. My great-uncle Fred taught me the ropes, but not the dead reckoning system using compass, landmarks, and coordinates of time and speed to chart your course. Nearly forty years later, still before the advent of GPS systems on most civilian boats, a couple of friends and I hatched the plan for a self-styled sailing retreat, and to qualify to charter the 36-foot Bavaria sloop and sail it ourselves, two of us had to pass a skills course that included dead reckoning navigation. My friend John and I signed on for the five-day course at sea and I still have those charts, still use them sometimes, though just for the fun of it; the boats today are equipped with GPS navigation and that's what we rely on. Which is fine as long as it works. But a few years ago, we set out for a short trip in a different boat, on unfamiliar waters, and our GPS failed. It was our memory of those dead reckoning skills and how to use them in the moment that enabled us to make our way safely to our destination.

Memory is the brain's own dead reckoning system. Whether you're navigating a waterway or a life passage, a challenge at home or work or school, or just want to reminisce about old times, pick up the right groceries, or show up when you said you would, how you do that relies on your brain's capacity to remember: to listen, learn, recall, process new information and evaluate and translate all of that into meaning and action. Alzheimer's gums up the works. In effect, it destroys the compass and coordinates of memory, eventually leaving the mind adrift at sea.

So often, when I would see patients with the mild or moderate cognitive impairment that brought them to a doctor's attention, they were impatient with their forgetfulness, discouraged or depressed by the sense that they were, however incrementally, mentally slipping away. They feared where it was leading, what they would lose next. They were especially fearful of losing their independence. The family members who accompanied them were often even more stricken. In addition to the practical consequences of their aging family member's needs, they also were already, in a way, losing the person they knew, or had known all along. Unmoored, all of them, in dark waters. The only certainty, the lone fixed point on the horizon was Alzheimer's itself and there was no comforting light there.

That beacon of hope lies in charting the neurological changes in the pre-symptomatic stage of Alzheimer's sooner, when evidence of the earliest changes to the neurological regions of memory can be detected in scans or tests, measured, monitored and, perhaps, treated to slow them down or support the brain's ability to provide backup or alternate neural networks. From the inside, observing our own mind at work, those earliest changes can be subtle and fleeting, even to a trained eye like mine. In many instances, in any single individual, some signs might easily be nothing more than symptoms of distractedness or memory slips brought on by excessive multitasking, overwork, poor sleep, chronic stress, deficiencies in diet or exercise, or other lifestyle factors. In my case, before I *was* a case, it would have been reasonable to assume that about myself. I was so consumed with growing work commitments, a growing family and growing community responsibilities that there was hardly room to track them in my day planner, much less make a mental note of every new name and phone number.

As 2013 approached, I took on expanded administrative responsibilities as director of the neurology resident training program at OHSU. It took a lot of effort to keep multiple balls in the air. I had to organize weekly lectures for the residents while giving several lectures myself. All fall I was consumed with reading about 200 applications from medical students applying to our program, organizing interviews with about 40 of those, and chairing the committee that made the final rankings for the national resident matching program to fill our 4 slots. I was also spending at least half my time seeing general neurology patients in clinic and supervising the neurology residents in their clinics and on the wards.

I relied on detailed to-do lists as well as copious notes, as most people do when multitasking in such circumstances, and things went well. But I began to feel that it seemed harder for me to manage than it should have been. By the beginning of 2013, I was beginning to have some symptoms that, as a neurologist, I recognized as mild cognitive impairment. I had trouble recalling names and occasional words – not uncommon for anyone my age, but I started to notice some issues with making plans and multitasking. I realized that I couldn't learn the phone number or address of my new office.

To see whether these concerns were anything more than the effects of normal aging, I arranged with a neurologist friend, a dementia specialist, to do some off-the-record cognitive testing with a computerized test. I actually did very well, but there was a caveat. On all but one of the cognitive domains tested, I scored above the 95th percentile. In other words, I did better than 95 percent of a normal cross-section of the population. However, on verbal memory I scored at the 50th percentile, exactly average. Verbal memory is memory that involves spoken or written words and ideas, and is involved in many tasks, including reading, writing, conversation, and recall of words and ideas. So, despite all of the cognitive tests being normal, there was a hint that all was not well with the parts of my brain responsible for verbal memory. The mild difficulties I was encountering mirrored the test scores.

If memory could be mapped like an island archipelago, much of what we casually think of as memory would be on the surface, above water, recognizable: formed memories around events, people, experiences, senses, emotions and feelings. Things we've done or learned, or ideas we've thought or talked about. Remembering to stop by the store to pick up milk on the way home, and then remembering when in the store to actually pick up the milk. Memory is an aspect of our mentality that allows us to recognize and revisit experience. But, as a neurological phenomenon, the brain's processes and neural networks for memory lie far below the waterline. In those hidden depths, when everything is working right, the currents and connections do their work unobstructed, unobserved, allowing smooth passage above. At that level, memory is enabling the brain to make the most basic connections that enable us to read and write, recognize a spoon and know how to use it, what to do with it, and recognize ourselves. But when something like Alzheimer's disrupts that flow, the effects eventually show up in observable changes in behavior and cognitive function.

More specifically, Alzheimer's doesn't just block the flow, it alters the neural archipelago of memory. So-called declarative memory – the memory of facts and events – is located in the temporal lobe and other parts of the cerebral cortex, whereas procedural memory – how to ride a bike or play the piano – is located deeper in the brain in the basal ganglia and cerebellum. Problems with declarative memory occur early in Alzheimer's, while procedural memory is usually not affected until late in the disease. People with very advanced Alzheimer's disease, unable to recognize family and sometimes unable to speak, can sometimes still play complex piano pieces from memory. For some reason, these circuits for procedural memory deep in the brain are not as vulnerable to the ravages of Alzheimer's as are the cortical regions located closer to the surface of the brain.

Declarative memory is further broken down into three components: immediate recall (like mental rehearsal of a phone number) lasts for a matter of seconds; memory for recent events lasts up to a few minutes; and long-term memory of distant events can potentially last for a lifetime. The hippocampus, a structure on the inner edge of the brain's temporal lobe, consolidates recent memory into long-term memory. Long-term memory is stored in various areas of the cerebral cortex.[1]

Location matters. Although, as we know now, olfactory centers in the brain are usually the first to be affected by

---

[1]   The classification of types of memory can be confusing. For example, some texts and papers use the terms *implicit* and *explicit* memory. Implicit memory is essentially the same as procedural memory, the memory for things that you do automatically, like riding a bike or playing a musical instrument. Explicit memory is the same as declarative memory – the memory for words, events from the past, and ideas.

Alzheimer's disease, most people don't notice a gradual impairment of their ability to smell. The hippocampus and its connections are the next to be damaged in most cases, resulting in impairment of recent memory and the ability to form new long-term memories. Memories of distant events that are already laid down usually are preserved until later in the disease.

Other cognitive domains are affected as Alzheimer's progresses. Language problems can occur early along with the memory issues. These include trouble thinking of the right word to say, saying the wrong word, reduced vocabulary, and poor comprehension. Visual–spatial impairment often follows soon after the onset of memory and language problems and may occasionally be the first symptom. This may result in misplacing things, getting lost, or having problems recognizing objects or even faces.

Problems with executive function are common relatively early in the disease and consist of trouble with motivation and making plans. The ability to multitask is lost. These activities are controlled in the prefrontal cortex, at the very front of the brain. Interestingly, the prefrontal cortex is one of the areas where amyloid plaques first appear in the brains of people who go on to have Alzheimer's disease (see Color Plate 1). As the disease progresses, there are usually difficulties with motor activities like using simple tools, dressing, feeding and other tasks, requiring increasing assistance from care-givers. In the middle and later stages, psychiatric symptoms can be an issue. These can include agitation, paranoia, hallucinations, and aggression.

By the beginning of 2013, by most standards I was still cognitively normal. My fund of neurological knowledge was robust and easily accessible. I was still able to teach effectively. Family life was still going full throttle. However, I was concerned by my nagging trouble with recall of names and words. Now I worried that they could be associated with the onset of Alzheimer's disease, especially knowing that my genes put me at high risk of having an Alzheimer's diagnosis by age 70. I was then 62. If I had been in almost any other job, I wouldn't have considered retiring, but in medicine there is no room for memory lapses or errors of judgment, and I felt it would be better to retire well before that risk became a reality. And so I did.

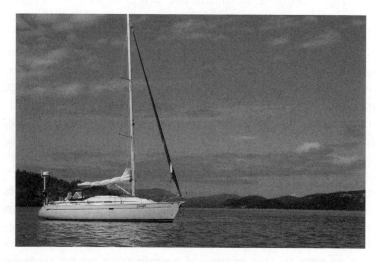

Escape is the Bavaria 36 sailboat that my friends John and Henry and I try to charter each summer. Here she is anchored at Hunter Bay on Lopez Island in Washington's San Juan Islands.

8 ORCAS
NONETHELESS

I had given no thought to retirement previously – I loved my work. The formality of early retirement upended any vision I might have conjured up of retiring at a ripe old age. Yet the abundance of caution that prompted me to retire from formal duties changed surprisingly little about the opportunities for me to contribute as a medical volunteer, where I could support on-site clinicians and patients, and consult with colleagues, locally and internationally. Nothing had substantially changed about my ability to teach – or to learn, for that matter – and in the year after I retired, I maintained a full slate of teaching and volunteer services. Little things came up from time to time, the occasional blanks recalling names and such. But I was able to continue my teaching trips to Tanzania, and to Ethiopia and the Congo. In Portland, I volunteered in a local free clinic providing primary care to visiting immigrants and uninsured Americans. In this setting, I had an experienced family doctor or internist available to supervise and inform my care of patients.

In some ways, these were the kinds of educational and volunteer service activities I might have imagined for my retirement years, but I accepted that the reason for my early retirement changed some of those options, and I grew more vigilant for any signs that might suggest early cognitive decline and the need to tailor my commitments further. About a year after retiring, as 2014 began and these mild incidents of lapses in recall continued, I arranged to see a dementia specialist for a formal cognitive assessment.

The results on that formal cognitive testing were normal, except, my neurologist noted, for delayed verbal
recall, which was slightly below average for age, which
meant that my memory for words and language was not
as good as it should have been. The evaluation summary
concluded that "the most appropriate diagnosis is subjec-
tive cognitive impairment, or mild cognitive impairment
(MCI) based on complaints only." That is to say, what struck
me as possible early symptoms of Alzheimer's didn't really
move the needle on a formal evaluation. I didn't even meet
any research criteria for MCI.

Although my cognitive function was still high by all
measures, I decided that, if even the earliest conditions for
neurodegenerative activity were developing in my brain –
so early that symptoms might still be years away – then now
was the time to find out, while there might be something
that could delay the progression of the disease. Once brain
cells are dead, then the horse is out of the barn; better to act
to protect or preserve what you've got while you've got it.
The more I knew now, the better. Given my circumstances
and my predilection for research, analyzing data and inter-
preting it in the context of patients' everyday experience of
symptoms, it felt natural to turn that clinical gaze more fully on myself. I would be my own longitudinal study of one.

It wasn't what I'd had in mind for this time in my life.
But an uninvited change of course sometimes delivers
in unexpected ways. Sailing had taught me that. At first
glance, it seems impossible that a sailboat can sail into
an oncoming wind. The physics of aerodynamics explains
how manipulating sails, speed and position can move you
forward on an angle into the wind. If your destination is
in the same direction as the source of the wind, it is necessary to come about, or tack, periodically to approach
the destination in a zig-zag fashion. Although the speed
you maintain toward your destination as the crow flies is
slower sailing into the wind, most sailors would agree that

this is the most thrilling and enjoyable point of sail. You have to pay attention to detail at every moment. The wind direction is changing, second by second, and to maintain maximum speed, fine tuning of the boat direction and sail trim has to be adjusted continuously. The boat is tilting, or heeling, and the apparent wind speed is high because it combines the actual wind speed and the added wind speed from the movement of the boat. If the water is rough, the spray hits you in the face, and the overall sense of speed, wind and spray can be exhilarating. By contrast, most sailors would agree that sailing directly downwind on a run is pretty boring. You may not feel the wind at all because the boat speed cancels out the wind speed. For the most part, sailing is not primarily about reaching a destination. It's all about the joy of getting there.

Often the joy isn't even about getting where you planned, but more about being where you are. A couple of years ago, on our annual August sailing trip, my friends and I were

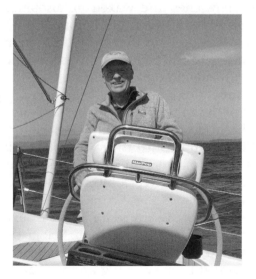

At the helm of *Escape*. Author's collection.

heading out from an island harbor to more open water for the day. The Salish Sea is prime whale-watching territory in the summer, and orca whales – actually a kind of dolphin – are a favorite. But they can also be elusive, and it's easy to spend a day out looking for them and never see one at all. We hoped to get lucky. There wasn't enough wind to sail, so we used the diesel engine to head for the Haro Strait, the large channel that separates Vancouver Island in British Columbia from the San Juan Islands in Washington State. The local pod of orcas is more often than not found somewhere near the Haro Strait. Within thirty minutes, the engine temperature alarm sounded, telling us the engine was overheating. We checked that there was water coming out of the exhaust pipe and there was. We checked the engine coolant level and it was OK. We let the engine cool down a bit and tried again. Within a few minutes, the alarm came on again. We called for a tow and settled in for the hour-and-a-half wait under the sun, sails still slack in the windless morning, drifting aimlessly. We made sandwiches and waxed philosophical, picking up where we'd left off the night before. We stared out at the quiet sea, watching for the towboat. Given the unlucky complications with the engine, we were resigned to a day now devoted to engine repair dockside.

Then, just about 100 yards away, a pod of orcas appeared – soaring out of the water in a brilliant flash and disappearing as quickly in clean dives, resurfacing again, and repeating the choreography until they were out of sight. There were eight or ten of them, and it was a spectacular sight. We were ecstatic, dumbstruck by our good luck.

After twenty years of these trips, I have found that the times you see the orcas are when you least expect them, not when you are trying to find them. You just stumble on them. We would have completely missed them that year if our engine had been working and we had headed out farther as planned.

When I think back to the years after I first retired, I'm reminded of that day on the water, stalled out and adrift for all practical purposes, our plans upended, but the day full of the memorably ordinary things of life. The gift of the orcas. The gift of time.

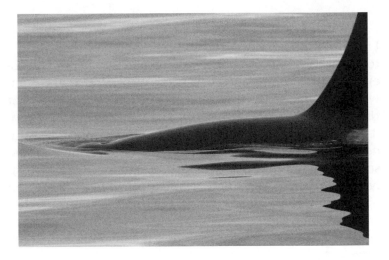

Orca.

9 MY BRAIN, MY SELF

I doubt I'm the only father of the bride who has written a toast for the rehearsal dinner, then worried about whether I'd be able to memorize it, tried, worried still and then written it out to have in my pocket just as backup. Not the only one who nervously patted his pocket to be sure it was there, then patted that pocket a few more times to double-check. Jokes about "senior moments" are a constant through-line among people my age. Who can honestly say they haven't blanked on a name, lost a list, forgotten where they put the car keys or, for that matter, forgotten why they interrupted what they were doing in one room to go to another, and remembered why only long after they gave up?

My new hypervigilance about my own "moments" might have seemed excessive at times. But, having just retired from a long career in brain science, suddenly I had unlimited time and access to study my own, and I was intrigued as well as motivated. I'd hoped to qualify as a research subject for new treatment options, get into some studies a.s.a.p. to put the brakes on any disease process that could be changed with treatment. My high scores meant I didn't qualify for clinical trials – not yet anyway. But I began building a case for it, documenting signs of cognitive impairment that would, I hoped, eventually expand the opportunity for people like me – with early signs and clearly at risk – to get into these studies. With that in mind, through the year ahead, I turned even closer attention to tracking my cognitive function for any signs of loss.

In many ways, the changes were imperceptible to others. I used lists and calendar notes more often – my private back-up system. Those worked, but I began to note other subtle stumbling blocks in cognitive function. Language was one. A public speaker, conference presenter and university lecturer, I'd taken for granted the ease I felt communicating this way. I'd spent most of my career, most of my days, in conversation with patients, colleagues and students, and had always enjoyed it, never felt burdened or stressed by the prospect. Now, I frequently would have to pause to find the word I wanted. I also was having trouble with comprehension at times, especially if I couldn't clearly hear every word that was said to me. I soon realized that I could no longer reliably extrapolate missing words from context. I continued to volunteer and travel, but this cognitive gap created new challenges that I couldn't fix with a list or sticky note. On my annual spring working trip to Tanzania, I found that I could no longer easily follow the medical conference – the morning report – in the hospital at the start of each day. It had always been a challenge in the past because most of the young doctors, although they spoke English, spoke softly with heavy accents, and the acoustics of the room were bad. But where I once had been able to adapt to that and follow along, now the conversation was garbled, unintelligible to me.

One day at home, I realized that I was getting worse at remembering names. I'd been blocked on the next-door neighbor's first name for several weeks. I could remember his last name and his wife's full name but not his. I was determined not to ask Lois because she got concerned if I admitted to too many memory lapses. Then two incidents of absent-mindedness in a single day disturbed me. Both were glitches in ordinary kitchen routines I'd done a million times. I always make the salad for dinner. That night I peeled the cucumber into the salad bowl instead of into the compost container next to the salad bowl. I didn't notice it at all until Lois asked quizzically why there was cucumber peel in the salad. She was good-natured about it. Then, unloading the dishwasher, I put a coffee mug on the shelf with my beer mugs. Not a big deal, but I have never done that before, and again I didn't recognize that I had done it until Lois pointed it out. As dementia advances and cognitive impairment worsens, one doesn't notice these little slips that one makes. But I was painfully cognizant of them. Lois often pointed out the memory lapses to help me focus and pay attention, but she was kind about it and would also help me laugh it off.

I stepped up the note-taking on myself, but then realized, when I'd go to review them, that gaps in the entries meant that I sometimes forgot to make any entries at all. *Note to self: remember to remember to make notes to self.*

None of this intruded on our good times, which were plentiful, with our older daughter's summer wedding to help plan, and our son and his wife expecting their first child soon after. And our saddest moment had nothing to do with Alzheimer's. We were devastated when our dog of nine years died suddenly, leaving us not only empty-nester parents, our kids now launched and on their own, but devoted dog-people bereft without a dog. In July, we embarked on a road trip to Northern California to help our younger daughter pack up for a move to graduate school back east, then celebrated my birthday – I was now 63 – and brought home a new puppy.

Lois and I had decided that, without kids around, we needed someone for both of us to care about and take care of. Jack was all that. The trouble was, I didn't realize I wasn't holding up my end of the caretaking bargain. Our house still bears evidence of his obsessive chewing in nearly every room on the ground floor. He chewed on the furniture, some of it several generations old; he chewed on baseboards, moldings, doors, and even the carved woodwork framing our fireplace. Jack's teething activity was particularly upsetting because he did it on my watch – Lois was busy with wedding planning and I was supposed to keep an eye on him while I worked at my desk nearby. But, absorbed in my work, I'd forget about Jack. This was new. I had always been a master of multitasking. More often now, when I put my attention on one thing, my awareness of other things going on around me dimmed. Jack was just being a puppy, but his behavior was showing me up. Lois mostly just took up the slack, not one to make people feel worse about mistakes when they're already beating themselves up for it.

Otherwise, it turned out to be something of a charmed summer. I relied on lists and a calendar to stay on task and it usually worked. Once I accidentally deleted a list on my phone and had some trouble reconstructing it, but managed. I didn't need to look at my notes to deliver that toast at our daughter's wedding. And when our son and daughter-in-law made us grandparents a couple of months later, I felt nothing but lucky again. Despite my concerns about mild cognitive impairment, when it came to calming a baby, apparently, I was something of a natural baby-whisperer, as Lois put it. I don't know where that capacity resides in the brain, but it felt like a bonus to me.

By November, there were some subtle slips in memory that I noted in my journal to share later with my doctor – I couldn't be sure anymore that I'd remember otherwise. I thought I detected a slight worsening in my ability to consolidate immediate memory into even short-term memory, like trying to remember a phone number long enough to write it down. My long-term memory was largely intact, although some holes were starting to appear. Like occasional events from the past that I just couldn't remember, even when Lois prompted me. ("Oh, you remember when we … don't you?" "Uh, nope.") Procedural memory seemed essentially normal – I could still drive, play the piano, and walk and move about normally. However, I suspected there might be some mild problems with executive function, possibly affecting my setting goals and following through. I found I

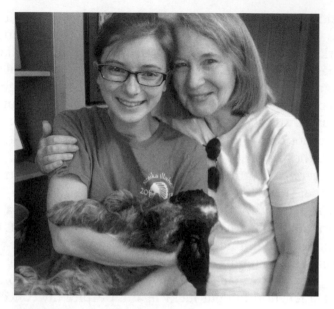

Meeting Jack for the first time.

had to write out a plan for the day when I first got up in the morning. Without that, I just couldn't stay on track to get anything accomplished. But I couldn't be sure whether this might instead be due to problems with short-term memory that have to do with not remembering the goal and plans. Either way, it was frustrating and worried me a little. I made a note of it. But I don't know how many times I *meant* to make a note of it before I actually followed through.

December brought an uptick in some mild problems with proprioception – the body awareness that lets you move smoothly from, say, the kitchen table to the kitchen sink, or shopping the aisles at the grocery store. I felt a little unsteady when I didn't have my glasses on, especially on tile floors; once on the carpet, I was fine. At the gym, I noticed that when I used the elliptical machine, I could only synchronize my breathing to my gait (which ordinarily you do naturally) if there were no other rhythmic sound around me. No music, no nothing. Usually at the gym, when I was on the elliptical, there was someone near me running on a treadmill and now my breathing always entrained to their gait, not my own. It was impossible for me to override this isolated glitch in my neural processing. When I'd run on a treadmill myself, I'd have no issues. If I rode a bicycling machine, I was able to synchronize my breathing with the cycles. My theory is that the sound of those machines, as mild as those sounds are, engage the neural pathways that connect sound to movement. The elliptical machine makes no sound. This suggests to me that pathways involving sound are intact but there may be some dysfunction in these proprioceptive pathways. Of course, I don't know yet whether people with normal proprioception also have this issue, but I suspect that they don't.

As the months passed, my file of notes grew fatter, and by the time we rang in the new year, it seemed to me that 2015 would likely be the year I would finally qualify – finally show enough cognitive impairment – for the research studies. Not everyone's idea of a happy new year thought, but for me it at least held the hope of finally getting some traction with medically based early treatment for what seemed likely to be early-stage Alzheimer's.

An early spring check-up with Dr. Rabinovici, my neurologist at UCSF, surprisingly showed my cognitive testing was unchanged from the year before. He noted one change: I scored high on the depression evaluation, which didn't surprise me at all. Virtually everyone who receives a diagnosis of Alzheimer's disease will suffer what doctors call reactive, or situational, depression. The diagnosis is, on the face of it, depressing. It's tough news to get. The future appears bleak. There is a real sense of loss. There is grieving. Even though I didn't yet have that diagnosis, I'm a neurologist, after all, and I knew what I knew: it was coming. My answers on the depression evaluation stated the obvious: Did I feel sad? Of course I felt sad. Did I feel discouraged about

the future? Of course I did, particularly given that I knew
about studies under way that might slow the progress of
this disease in its early stages, but my cognitive impairment
wasn't "bad enough" to qualify for them. So I was witness-
ing my own neurodegeneration in slow motion, and adding
to my frustration was the fact that the debate about how
to formally classify or even identify early-stage Alzheimer's
stood between me and potential new treatments.

Dr. Rabinovici talked with me about participating in a
longitudinal study of patients at risk for Alzheimer's that
he had under way, but there were delays. I couldn't help
but think of all the people much like myself – millions –
who could be in the very earliest stages of neurological
changes that set the stage for Alzheimer's, and how much
could be learned by identifying that stage, studying it, and
advancing the science and medical treatments to make a
significant difference in someone's life for, well, the rest
of their life.

But I knew the day for that diagnosis would come, and
this was no time to take a wait-and-see approach. There
was too much at stake. I had already decided some months
back that even if my cognitive scores continued to be
high – too high for me to qualify for the research studies – I could still take steps on my own to start an aggressive regimen of diet, exercise and other activities that have
been shown to build cognitive resilience and slow the progression of Alzheimer's. That research is extensive and the
findings clear. Always, as a doctor, one's aim is not only
to treat or to manage illness, but to do everything possible to prevent it. For now, there were definite preventive
steps I could move ahead with on my own. Actual prevention might not be possible, but if preventive steps could
provide a protective effect – slow the speed or spread of
the neurodegeneration – that was the point.

So I self-prescribed what I would have suggested to my
patients in the same position. I adopted a strategic regimen

of more exercise, with more of it aerobic; a modified Mediterranean diet called the MIND diet, with special emphasis on brain-healthy foods; and everyday activities that kept me socially active and mentally stimulated: crossword puzzles once or twice daily, reading six to ten books per month. I had a little trouble remembering what I'd read a few days later, but it helped to tell Lois about what I was reading – it firmed up my memory. Fortunately, she's a voracious reader herself, and she was a good sport about it.

In fact, Lois was very supportive of this whole new workout regimen of mine. She was a reliable thumbs-up for all of my exercise and outdoor activities – from my workouts and the neighborhood gym to my long walks with Jack and my occasional day trips to spend time with a few old friends boating on the Columbia River. She eventually confessed that she was grateful for what she called her "solitary splendor" – being able to reclaim some time by herself to keep up with her own interests and other activities. We are two introverts, both of us on the quiet, bookish side, but we do enjoy each other's company and conversation. Apparently, however, the challenge of having a spouse retire and suddenly be around the house all the time is a thing. Especially when you're accustomed to long days on your own schedule, with your own commitments, much of it in your own company or in phone and texting conversations with your adult kids, friends and colleagues, and improvisational conversations with your dog.

I could hardly complain. In our conversations, I would frequently have to ask Lois to repeat what she had said because I had missed the first few words and couldn't make sense of those words I had heard. This also was becoming a particular problem in groups when several people were speaking at once, and, whether the group was family or friends around the dining room table, a class of my students or colleagues at the medical school, or in morning rounds, it was unnerving for me to have to strain to hear what people were saying. And the truth was, it didn't work.

Lois is an expert at the art of one step at a time, whether it's on a mountain trek, a family wedding, or this early-stage Alzheimer's journey. From her earlier career as a librarian, then in marriage, motherhood, the role of family event planner and rememberer of all birthdays and anniversaries, through the steady stream of books she reads, the puzzles she starts *and* finishes, and the countless creative paths she pursues – quilting, knitting – and in the tapestry of family life in which her hand is always present, she has the remarkable capacity to keep the big picture and the smallest details in focus; I cannot imagine how all that would look on an MRI scan. But I do know what Alzheimer's looks like on a brain scan, and I would soon be looking for those signature details on my own.

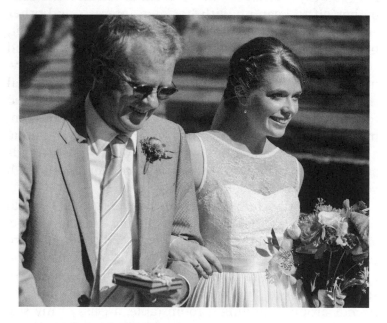

Father of the bride. Photo by Erin Grace Porozni.

10 THE REVEAL

Ordinarily – or a few years ago, at least – I would have walked into a conference room with thirty colleagues around the table and been prepared either to present or to consult on a case. This day was different. Today, I was the case.

The brain-imaging study that brought me to San Francisco in September 2015, more than two years after my retirement, would establish a baseline for measuring my cognitive loss going forward. Dr. Gil Rabinovici had invited me to take part in a long-term brain-imaging study for subjects at risk for Alzheimer's disease. This work-up involved two PET scans, a high-resolution MRI, and two days of cognitive testing. One of the PET scans could detect the abnormal amyloid protein found in plaques, which are seen up to twenty years before onset of cognitive impairment. The other PET scan could detect the abnormal tau protein found in the neurofibrillary tangles of Alzheimer's disease. After four days of scans and extensive cognitive testing, on the fifth day I met with the research and clinical team for the reveal – the medical team version of the "family conference" – to go over the results of the studies.

All eyes were on the presentation screen, much as mine had been since the first time I'd seen a scanned image of a living human brain nearly forty years ago in medical school. I vividly remember the first time I saw a real-time image of a living human brain. The hospital had just purchased an

EMI scanner.[1] This would have been in 1977 or 1978, and, prior to that advancement, there was almost no ability to see the brain during life – except, of course, during surgery. I was in medical school and X-rays showed the bones of the skull, and calcium in the pineal gland often made it visible on an X-ray, making it possible to see whether there was any gross asymmetry to the brain, but there was no routine way to actually see the brain tissue. It seemed like magic to have a true image, a "slice" through the human brain. The pixel size was enormous by modern standards, about 3 × 3 mm, so the image looked almost like a patchwork quilt or impressionist painting. By contrast, modern CT scanners have pixels that are about 0.5 × 0.5 mm. It still was fantastic. Primitive as the pixel size was at that time, the image was remarkable. That first scan I saw was of the brain of a patient who had recently had a stroke. The patient was still in the scanner and we could see the image of the dark area within the brain that was caused by the stroke. In the 1980s, MRI scans arrived and provided even more detail of normal and abnormal brain structures, but the magic of seeing that first CT image stays with me still. Imaging today has advanced so much, and I'm still amazed by the way it reveals the reality of the functioning brain in such rich detail: the illustrated brain.

Now the illustrated brain on the scan was mine.

Dr. Rabinovici, as the research study director, introduced me to everyone around the table: psychologists, neurologists and technicians who had been doing the testing, and an assortment of others whose research focus or medical training involved dementia. He then asked, as a formal part of the patient interview, how I would feel if the scans

[1]   The British company EMI was perhaps best known as the Beatles' first recording company, but EMI was also the first company to sell a CT scanner. "CT" stands for "computerized tomography." The first CT scans were therefore called "EMI scans," but as other companies entered the field, the name was forever changed to "CT scan."

were abnormal, indicating that I had the brain pathology of Alzheimer's disease. I'd come to consider Dr. Rabinovici as something of a colleague, as we'd often discuss clinical interests outside the scope of my personal participation in the study. I knew that his question was standard. I just hadn't experienced it from the patient's side of the table before. I'd never sat with a group of colleagues gathered to talk about *my* brain, *my* cognition and *my* diagnosis.

"I have no doubt that's what the scans are going to show," I said, "given the combination of my mild cognitive impairment and my two copies of the APOE-4 gene. I'd be very surprised if they turned out to be normal and would have to look elsewhere for the cause for my cognitive issues." But there would be no need for that.

Dr. Rabinovici then proceeded to show the scans in detail, and, as expected, they were all abnormal. Perhaps surprisingly, I actually felt a sense of relief. Everything finally made sense. And the scans themselves were, just objectively speaking, beautiful in the way brain scans are to me.

There they were, the unmistakable tell-tale signs of Alzheimer's. The amyloid PET scan showed a moderate amount of beta-amyloid in the frontal lobes and lesser amounts in the temporal, parietal and occipital lobes. The most intense abnormality was in the prefrontal cortex, which is involved in executive function, and, as it happened, two other brain areas which are involved in processing olfactory information. I was fascinated to see, in this anatomical image of my brain, the correlation of the loss of smell to brain changes that now appeared to have been the harbinger of my Alzheimer's disease (Color Plate 1). The tau PET scan showed the beginnings of abnormal tau, primarily in the temporal lobes, as shown in Color Plate 2.

The hippocampus is the area of the brain where recent memory is converted to long-term memory and is one of the first parts of the brain to be affected in Alzheimer's disease, so it wasn't surprising to see the spreading abnormal tau in my case. The MRI scan showed moderate atrophy, or wasting away, of the medial portion of the temporal lobes, especially in the left hippocampus. There was also mild to moderate enlargement of the ventricles, the cavities within the brain that contain cerebrospinal fluid. This indicates the generalized wasting away caused by death of nerve cells.

At the conference table presentation that day, a small detail on the amyloid PET scan caught my eye, and I asked Dr. Rabinovici to enlarge it for us to examine more closely. It was the area of the scan that included the olfactory centers. He zoomed in on it for us all to study, and, sure enough, there was evidence of amyloid in the piriform cortex and medial portion of the orbitofrontal cortex, both important centers for processing of olfactory information in the brain. My loss of smell and the illusory odors of baking bread had started about eight years before, and here, finally, appeared to be the tangible proof of a connection. This observable connection on a PET scan between amyloid concentration and olfactory centers wasn't something that had been reported in the literature before, so far as we knew, and the novel discovery of it here created a bit of a buzz in the room. For that moment, we were just a couple of dozen scientists around a big table, studying scans, and we thought it was pretty cool. As a scientist, there's nothing quite like the thrill of discovery. Even if it was my own brain on the screen.

That thrill of discovery is not the case for most patients. More often it's a sobering, or sometimes frightening, epiphany. Among my patients, reviewing the results of tests and scans that confirmed signs of Alzheimer's got mixed reviews. Some said the information was clarifying: they weren't happy to hear it, but it helped ground their thinking about next steps in a treatment plan we would develop together. Others who came to see me were there at the urging of someone else – sometimes a family mem-

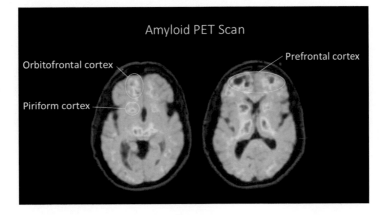

Color plate 1: This is my amyloid PET scan in September 2015, performed as part of a research study. This particular amyloid radiotracer is not yet approved for clinical use. Beta-amyloid shows up as yellow, orange and red color, with red being the most intense concentration. The two horizontal slices through my brain are about a half-inch apart and show beta-amyloid accumulation in the prefrontal cortex (executive action) and the orbitofrontal and piriform cortex (both involved in olfactory processing). This would be a typical PET scan of someone with early-stage Alzheimer's disease. Courtesy of Dr. Gil Rabinovici, UCSF Memory and Aging Center.

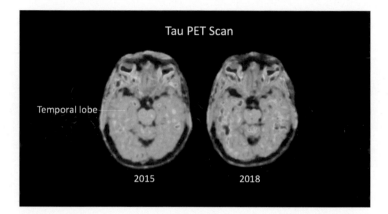

Color plate 2: These are two tau PET scans three years apart, through the same horizontal slice of my temporal lobes. This investigational tau radiotracer has just recently been approved for clinical use. My imaging was performed for research purposes only. The first scan shows the beginnings of tau deposition seen as yellow, orange and red colors, primarily in the temporal lobes. (The intense red seen in the eyes is only an imaging artifact.) Three years later, the tau signal is more intense and has spread on both sides farther back into the temporal lobes, more so on the left. Courtesy of Dr. Gil Rabinovici, UCSF Memory and Aging Center.

ber, friend or perhaps a supervisor at work – and often what they wanted most of all was to avoid a formal diagnosis of dementia. In some cases, they feared losing their job and livelihood. In others, the specter of a dementia diagnosis threatened to upend their sense of themselves and their standing in their profession, family or community. The positive potential of any treatment was often overshadowed by their fears. The problem in the past was that we didn't recognize the disease until people were already in the moderate to late stages of it. It didn't help that, back when I first started practicing in the early 1990s, there was nothing we could do. There were no drugs, we didn't know anything about lifestyle changes – and I hated that we were so helpless to do anything about it. It was the same as cancer had been twenty years before that. Nobody talked about it. Many people didn't want to know.

Over those years, in my practice I saw every kind of response to the clinical evidence of a neurological concern, especially dementia. Now it was my turn to receive the news. I'd been shocked to first discover my APOE-4 risk factor in the genealogy report, but by now my shock had subsided and I'd resorted to my default setting, which is to focus on the science and research, analyzing all relevant evidence and credible theories. I understand that this is in part a coping mechanism to manage what would otherwise perhaps be emotionally overwhelming. So, focusing on the granular details grounds me in the scientific literature, which is a comfort zone for me, and it gives me a toehold in the current research and data that my doctors will be studying as well. Everybody processes unsettling news in their own way, at their own pace. But eventually the meaningful next step is to move on to sorting through the particulars of the situation, clinical and practical factors, because that process can ground us. It can be empowering as choices arise and decisions can be made. It beats surrendering to despair.

The rest of my work-up held no real surprises, but it did raise one question. The evidence in the imaging studies was all consistent with early-stage Alzheimer's disease. And yet my cognitive studies, for the most part, continued to look pretty good, still in the MCI range – better than what would be expected looking at those images. This apparent discrepancy wasn't unique to me; it has been found in others, though most often in post-mortem examinations of the brain, at the end of a life in which they had not shown symptoms of Alzheimer's despite the presence of the tell-tale plaques and tangles there in the brain.

One explanation for the discrepancy, specific to me because of my long years as a neurologist, was that I'd cheated on the test – or my brain had. I had at least some familiarity with most of the cognitive tests I was given because I'd given the tests to patients on an almost daily basis for many years. I knew most of the answers, and when I didn't know the answers, I knew how to derive them. I wasn't trying to beat the test, but I couldn't just command my brain to un-know the way it has learned to problem-solve as needed in these tests.

Another theory suggested that lifetime habits of study and stretching to learn, and other stimulating cognitive activity, contribute to so-called cognitive reserve, a kind of brain bank of neural cells or networks that provided backup, or created resilience, that might be keeping my cognitive functioning high despite the presence of brain atrophy and accumulations of plaques and tangles normally seen in mild to moderate Alzheimer's disease.

Whatever was responsible for my encouraging cognitive capacity at the present, I saw it as an opportunity I needed to seize, to learn more about what I could do – and what medical science might be able to do – to slow the progress of the disease and amp up my brain's defenses against it before it was too late.

11 COGNITIVE RESERVE AND RESILIENCY: BRAIN CELLS IN THE BANK

I spend much of my day reading science – updates on clinical studies, current journals, and deep dives into the growing scientific literature on the many facets of neuro-degenerative disease, dementia, Alzheimer's disease and, specifically, early-stage Alzheimer's. I also read spy novels and work crosswords throughout the day as if my life depended on it. In a way, it does.

The Holy Grail of Alzheimer's research is the search for a treatment that can halt the underlying disease process. A drug, a procedure, some sophisticated treatment regimen that, in medicine, we call a disease-modifying intervention. While nothing has proved reliably effective in clinical trials so far, a lot has been learned about what goes on in the brain during the disease process. The role of cognitive reserve and resiliency is something of a wild card – it's not fully understood – but it is emerging as a promising factor in the brain's capacity to forestall the effects of Alzheimer's for a longer period without significant symptoms. For those of us with early-stage Alzheimer's, it may offer a potential reprieve from the otherwise steady erosion of our faculties by the neurodegenerative disease process.

Although not a medical cure, cognitive reserve may be life-saving in a different way: helping preserve the life of the mind as the brain itself is under siege. Pressing alternate neural pathways into service or forging new ones, this reserve acts something like a backup generator to keep the lights on when the main power source is failing. This isn't magical thinking. Neuroscience has established that the resilient brain can create new connections and pathways for circuitry that has been damaged by disease or injury. It happens in some cases of stroke and a range of other types of brain damage.

Dr. Yaakov Stern was one of the first proponents of the concept of cognitive reserve, which he described as a neurological process in which "the brain actively attempts to cope with brain damage by using pre-existing cognitive processing approaches or by enlisting compensatory approaches." Someone with high cognitive reserve would be better able to cope with brain damage than someone whose cognitive reserve is lower, he held. Further, he noted in 2012, evidence suggested that it wasn't brain size (bigger brain, more neurons) that determined cognitive reserve. The extent of cognitive reserve differed for each person, he said, evidenced in the way that the same amount of brain damage has "different effects on different people, even when brain size is held constant." The relevant variable, he concluded, was brain function, not brain size [1].

Some things can compromise cognitive reserve. The two best studied of these are head injury and stroke. Since both of these often occur together in dementia, they could be a factor in causing or adding to cognitive impairment. This is the reason that reducing stroke risk with good blood pressure control, a heart-healthy diet, and good management of diabetes are all recommended tools in slowing the progression of Alzheimer's disease.

The study of cognitive reserve has continued to gain momentum in recent years, especially as findings have emerged from longitudinal studies of aging, the brain and neurodegenerative diseases. With the advent of high-resolution imaging that can show the atrophy in regions of the Alzheimer's brain, the concept of cognitive reserve has been further refined. A recent study reported in *JAMA Neurology* showed that high cognitive reserve, as measured by education and high baseline intelligence, *does not* protect from tau-associated brain atrophy, but it *does* lead to a delay in cognitive impairment, postponing the onset of the symptoms of Alzheimer's disease [2]. In other words, cognitive reserve does not reduce the tau-mediated brain damage of Alzheimer's, but it seems to provide cognitive resilience to the effects of this damage. And, in a study reported in *JAMANetwork*, researchers found that better cognition measured during high school was associated with decreased odds of dementia later in life [3]. In an editorial commenting on this paper, Dr. Tom Russ called for interventional research into improving cognitive reserve early in life as a tool to decreasing the risk of getting Alzheimer's:

> *[G]iven that we have a plausible mechanism – cognitive reserve – we now need to consider interventional research. The International Federation on Aging Copenhagen Summit on cognitive reserve in 2017 highlighted a number of factors that could potentially influence cognitive reserve, including modifiable health factors, education, social support, positive affect, stimulating activities and/or novel experiences, and cognitive training (http://www.ifa-copenhagensummit.com/). Not all of these are modifiable, and of those that are, not all are modifiable later in life, but the potential of intervening at many different stages of the life course to improve one – or ideally multiple – of these factors is there. If, as a result, cognitive reserve could be modified before the clinical onset of dementia (even if Alzheimer disease were present in the brain), this may delay the onset of these clinical symptoms which would, in turn, reduce the number of people affected by dementia worldwide. Given the growing global public health burden of dementia, this is a vital question. [4]*

These findings strongly support Dr. Stern's model of cognitive reserve and suggest that the apparent resilience is not due to more brain cells or protection from brain cell loss. Rather, it is likely due to richer connections between those neurons that we all have.

In Alzheimer's specifically, it turns out that the characteristic plaques and tangles appear in both groups – those with high cognitive reserve and those with low cognitive reserve – at about the same time and at about the same rate. The important distinction, according to Stern's model, is that the onset of cognitive impairment occurs later in people with high cognitive reserve.

Once people with high reserve start to get cognitive impairment, the trajectory toward the late stage of the disease is much more rapid. Put simply, everyone who

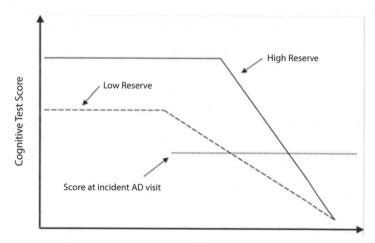

According to Stern's model, people with low cognitive reserve have lower cognitive test scores than those with high reserve, even before any Alzheimer's pathology begins. In both groups, neuropathology starts years before the beginning of cognitive impairment, and people with low cognitive reserve start having further decrease in cognitive ability several years before those with high reserve. Eventually, once those with high reserve start to have decreased cognition, they progress more rapidly and "catch up" with the low reserve group [1]. AD, Alzheimer's disease.

is going to get Alzheimer's disease gets pathology in the brain at about the same time, and they probably will die of the disease at about the same time, but those with high cognitive reserve will have better cognitive function longer – a delay in the start of the first cognitive symptoms – before the loss then progresses more rapidly. Cognitive reserve can buy you more quality time.

I'm confronting the prospect of that dramatic drop sometime ahead, but my interest right now is in extending the promising plateau any way I can. What can I do? Where does cognitive reserve come from? Are we just born with it or is it something that we can cultivate through life? No one really knows, but it is likely that the answer is a little of both. Our genetic make-up may play a part in our ultimate intelligence and cognitive reserve, but life-long learning, education and exercise probably play even larger roles. Stern summarized research findings that compared factors associated with less and more cognitive reserve, and identified the activities that seemed to result in greater cognitive reserve as follows:

1 Greater education: Those with less than eight years of schooling have twice the risk of developing dementia compared to those with more education.
2 Occupational achievement: Those with so-called lower occupational achievement (unskilled/semiskilled, skilled trade or craft, and clerical/office worker) also had a two-fold increase in risk of developing dementia compared to those with high occupational achievement (manager business/government and professional/technical).
3 Leisure activity: Subjects were asked about their participation in thirteen leisure activities in the previous month. These might include knitting or music or other hobby, walking for pleasure or on an excursion, visiting friends or relatives, being

visited by relatives or friends, physical conditioning, going to movies or restaurants or sporting events, reading magazines or newspapers or books, watching television or listening to the radio, doing unpaid community volunteer work, playing cards or games or bingo, going to a club or center, going to classes, and going to religious services. Those who participated in more than six of these leisure activities had about one-third less chance of developing dementia going forward.

A remarkable longitudinal study begun nearly thirty years ago, long before Stern's findings, found something similar. In the so-called Nun Study [5], researchers began tracking cognitive health and decline in a group of more than 300 members of the School Sisters of Notre Dame, an order of American Roman Catholic nuns in Minnesota. The nuns volunteered to participate in regular health assessments, and had cognitive and other tests done yearly. Their brains were examined after death. The Nun Study cohort eventually grew to include nearly 700 sisters of that Order, and in the three decades since it began, scientists have continued to parse the data and discover new insights about cognitive reserve and dementia, including how cognitive and linguistic abilities, in particular, appear to factor into Alzheimer's and other types of dementia. All the nuns had written autobiographical essays when entering the Order in their twenties, allowing a retrospective assessment of writing skills as young adults. From all of this, researchers found that the most highly educated and the most articulate writers were least likely to develop cognitive impairment, despite their APOE-4 status, suggesting a correlation with cognitive reserve that is largely accepted today.

As for my own cognitive reserve, I can't know how much might have been banked earlier in my life, but I'm encouraged and newly appreciative when I think about the way my parents supported my curiosity, creativity and critical thinking growing up. On an imaginary spreadsheet of cognitive reserve from my childhood, I see the hours spent with my father building toys and gadgets from scratch, creating fantastical (to me at a young age) experiments mostly centered around electricity and chemical reactions, and later going together to weekly public science lectures given by professors at a nearby university. I hear the hours with my mother at the piano, first listening as she played Beethoven, Bach, Rachmaninoff, and later studying under her watchful eye.

There's no way yet to measure cognitive reserve, no way for me to check mine to see whether my present steady diet of crosswords, reading and other stimulating pursuits is actually nudging the needle upward on my cognitive reserve or resiliency. But it reminds me a little of the satisfying feedback from the smartphone/exercise clinical trial that tracks my data as I workout. Although I can't see the data that shows a brain boost in cognitive reserve from a good book or game of scrabble, I can feel it. And I'm willing to keep up the experiment.

Chapter-references

1   Stern Y. Cognitive reserve in ageing and Alzheimer's disease. *Lancet Neurology* 2012; 11: 1006–1012; https:// doi.org/10.1016/S1474-4422(12)70191-96 (public access version available at www.ncbi.nlm.nih.gov/pmc/ articles/PMC3507991).

2   Xu H, Yang R, Qi X, *et al.* Association of lifespan cognitive reserve indicator with dementia risk in the presence of brain pathologies. *JAMA Neurology* 2019; 76:1184–1191; https://doi.org/10.1001/ jamaneurol.2019.2455 (public access version available at www.ncbi.nlm.nih.gov/pmc/articles/PMC6628596).

3 Huang AR, Strombotne KL, Horner EM, Lapham SJ. Adolescent cognitive aptitudes and later-in-life Alzheimer disease and related disorders. *JAMA Network Open* 2018; 1(5):e181726; https://doi.org/10.1001/jamanetworkopen.2018.1726.

4 Russ T. Intelligence, cognitive reserve, and dementia: time for intervention? *JAMA Network Open* 2018; 1(5):e181724; https://doi.org/10.1001/jamanetworkopen.2018.1724.

5 Snowden D. *Aging with Grace: What the Nun Study Teaches Us About Leading Longer, Healthier, and More Meaningful Lives*. Bantam Books, 2001.

12 MY EXPERIMENTAL LIFE

Headlines make scientific breakthroughs seem sudden, but, in truth, the real advancement of science is more like the construction of a pyramid. Each block of the pyramid represents a hypothesis that attempts to explain an observation in nature that has been tested experimentally. Depending on the results of the experiment, the hypothesis is either confirmed, revised and tested again, or rejected. Each block adds to a new layer of the pyramid, each layer built on those below. No single study is likely to crack the code for an immediate Alzheimer's cure, but each one contributes to our understanding in ways that I am confident will eventually lead to more effective treatment and prevention. Even if it's not in time for me.

Clinical trials are the bricks and mortar of medical science, and if having Alzheimer's means I've had to step away from any professional involvement with them, it also opened up a new opportunity to stay involved. Now I can be a subject, participate in clinical trials as a patient. That appeals to me.

The number of clinical trials for drugs and other ways to stop, slow or prevent neurodegenerative diseases has increased dramatically in recent years. As I write, there are 3,075 clinical trials under way or recently ended related to Alzheimer's, including some that are focused on aspects of early-stage Alzheimer's. The clinical trials are diverse. Some are for medical devices like deep brain stimulation and ultrasound for opening the protective blood–brain barrier. Some are for testing new biomarkers, and some are for diets and other lifestyle changes. But most are for new medications, including antibodies to remove beta-amyloid or tau, enzyme inhibitors that block the synthesis of beta-amyloid, gene modifiers, stem-cell derivatives and many others. Existing drugs are also being investigated with an eye to repurposing medications for inflammation, diabetes and other disorders that may influence the growth of Alzheimer's plaques and tangles.

More research is under way to improve methods to predict who will get the dementia of Alzheimer's disease before cognitive symptoms emerge. Most of the early work has been with markers for brain amyloid, the role of which in Alzheimer's is not fully understood. About 20 percent of elderly people have amyloid that shows up on their PET scans yet they are cognitively normal, and they have no MRI or FDG-PET[1] evidence of neurodegeneration [1]. So not everyone with amyloid in the brain will get clinical Alzheimer's disease before they die. Increasing evidence suggests that tau may be the more important marker to study. A recent report shows that the areas of tau seen on a PET scan predict where future brain atrophy will occur, whereas areas of amyloid seen on PET are not predictive [2]. Within a few years, it's likely that combinations of biomarkers – perhaps some not yet discovered – may prove to be useful predictors of Alzheimer's in the pre-symptomatic stage, when treatment has the best chance to work.

In the meantime, there's work to be done, and I'm able and willing to volunteer for it. Over the past five years, I've been screened for five clinical trials and was accepted into four of them. The one that wouldn't take me was a Phase

---

[1] Fluorodeoxyglucose PET scans are a measure of metabolic activity in the brain (and elsewhere). Regions of the brain showing decreased signal on an FDG-PET scan are associated with decreased metabolic activity and indicate possible neurodegeneration. FDG-PET is neither as specific nor as sensitive as amyloid PET for detecting evidence of Alzheimer's disease.

3 study of a monoclonal antibody (an antibody produced in a lab) that targets the abnormal tau protein that is the main component of the neurofibrillary tangles found in brains of people with Alzheimer's disease. At the time I applied to enter that study, I was deemed cognitively just a little too good to qualify. The other trials have been mostly easy and interesting, ranging from the longitudinal neuro-imaging study that first found the evidence of early-stage Alzheimer's in my brain, to a study that measures the immediate effects of exercise on cognition, and another looking for cognitive-enhancing properties in a botanical compound.

The single exception was a different Phase 3 trial of a promising monoclonal antibody that acts as a plaque-buster, targeting the beta-amyloid that forms the Alzheimer's plaques between brain cells. The stages in the development of any potential new pharmaceutical start with preclinical studies in animals to demonstrate effectiveness and probable safety, then progress through the three-phase process as they repeatedly prove safe and effective for humans. Phase 3 is the most advanced trial before a product or treatment that performs well is approved by the US Food and Drug Administration and made available for clinical use.

In March 2016, I entered a Phase 3 clinical trial of the antibody called aducanumab. The Phase 1 trial of this drug had looked very promising, effectively removing amyloid plaques and resulting in a trend toward slowing cognitive impairment [3]. Several similar anti-amyloid drugs had previously failed in Phase 3 trials, but there were several encouraging things about aducanumab that intrigued me. First, aducanumab was based on a naturally occurring antibody found in the blood of elderly people who did not have any cognitive impairment. In other words, despite being in their eighties and nineties, they had no symptoms of Alzheimer's disease. This antibody bound strongly to beta-amyloid, and researchers hypothesized that its anti-amyloid clearing action was responsible, at least in part, for the cognitive well-being of these elderly individuals.

Second, side effects appeared minimal. The only common side effects were headaches and, at higher doses, an odd swelling in parts of the brain, which usually caused no symptoms. Sometimes the swelling occurred along with tiny areas of bleeding into the brain. Because these could be detected on MRI scans, they were called Amyloid Related Imaging Abnormalities, or ARIA. Whenever ARIA were detected on scans during trials of anti-amyloid drugs, the medication was stopped until the imaging abnormality resolved. Then the medication could usually be restarted without the problem occurring again. Most of the subjects who developed ARIA had no symptoms at all – the ARIA were discovered in the periodic brain scans used to monitor effects for the duration of the clinical trial. Still, there was concern that ARIA could represent a potentially severe side effect, so in the early trials, dosages of these anti-amyloid antibodies were limited to minimize the chance of producing ARIA.

That was about to change. A much more aggressive dosing strategy was being used for aducanumab, especially in the Phase 3 trial. I thought this was a good idea. Since ARIA didn't seem to be too dangerous, it made sense to try higher doses of the drug. Finally, and most appealing, the results of the earlier Phase 1 trial looked very encouraging. Subjects receiving aducanumab had a marked reduction in brain amyloid as measured by PET, and there was a trend toward improved cognition. These results had been so strong that the pharmaceutical company was allowed to skip the usual Phase 2 trial and go directly to a Phase 3 trial. With the risk–benefit ratio strongly weighted toward potential benefit, I felt I had nothing to lose.

After a battery of baseline cognitive tests, a high-resolution MRI, and another amyloid PET scan, I received my first of eighteen monthly infusions. This was a double-blind study, meaning that neither I nor the study doctors and infusion nurses knew whether I was receiving a placebo or one of two doses of aducanumab. The test infusion was given intravenously over one hour while I was closely monitored for side effects. I had absolutely no side effects, not even headaches. This made me think that I was probably getting placebo, but I really didn't know.

Every month or two, I had MRI scans to check for ARIA but none were found during the double-blind stage. I got into a routine of once or twice a month getting up at 4 a.m. to catch the 6:30 a.m. flight from Portland to San Francisco, taking the BART train and MUNI tram to the UCSF campus at Mission Bay and usually arriving in time to get a cappuccino and breakfast at my favorite coffee shop two blocks from campus before my infusion at 11 a.m. I would get a late afternoon or early evening flight home. At the end of eighteen months, I had another battery of cognitive tests and another amyloid PET scan. I then started the optional two-year extension phase of the study. During this period, all volunteers received active aducanumab. None received placebo. At this point, I was almost sure I had been in the placebo arm of the double-blind phase of the trial, so I was excited to know that now I'd be taking the real drug.

Exciting in some ways, it was also a difficult time in others. The clinical trial's rigid schedule of drug infusions and evaluations, all in San Francisco, took priority over everything and everyone else in our family orbit. Concern for me and my health, and the risks involved in a drug study, as well as my traveling there alone for some of the checkups, were no small worry for Lois and the kids. My routine of pre-dawn departures and late-night returns upended other routines at home or made me inaccessible in ways that Lois was left to contend with.

The study required Lois to accompany me at regular intervals to answer routine questions about her observations of me in our everyday environment. To do so required an overnight stay so we could be there at their early start time. And that meant that we had to board Jack at a kennel for a night, sometimes two, depending on return flights. All of this required that Lois reorganize her own schedule of commitments or miss some, which she wouldn't have minded doing if her presence there had felt necessary at all. She felt that the rote questions that they asked her every time – *Can he tie his shoes? Can he operate the microwave?* – could easily have been answered in a phone or online format. Most important, she felt they ignored the subtler symptoms the study might have charted through this very early-stage situation. Instead, it skipped ahead to symptoms associated with more advanced cognitive impairment. At least my part in the study was interesting; hers was frustrating and I could understand why. It wasn't that she didn't want to contribute, but she felt the questions weren't designed to get at the reality of someone with *early-stage* Alzheimer's and only mild cognitive impairment, as opposed to the more advanced stages of the disease which are more commonly diagnosed. Lois has endless patience for many things, but not for what she considers limited efforts when it comes to digging for important information. Perhaps with greater attention to early-stage Alzheimer's in the field, the research tools will eventually be calibrated to learn even more about how the disease presents and progresses, and how to effectively intervene earlier.

When a Phase 3 clinical trial goes poorly or raises significant new concerns about patient safety, the project pushes pause on an extension phase since the drug isn't performing as expected or poses newly understood risks for new participants. However, in practical terms, when the extension phase moves ahead, it's because things look promising. Nothing guarantees that the extension phase of a study will end with a breakthrough. No one really knows for sure what the extended study will show. But, in a larger sense, in the broad sweep of history in medical science, every breakthrough is preceded by successful clinical trials. That turning point only becomes clear in retrospect, of course, but, as a research scientist, a neurologist and now an Alzheimer's patient, the turning point was where I wanted to be.

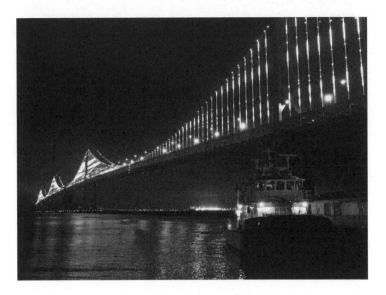

I took this photo of San Francisco's Bay Bridge during one of our multi-day visits to the UCSF Memory and Aging Center.

Chapter-references

1 Jack CR, Wiste HJ, Weigand SD, *et al.* Age-specific population frequencies of cerebral β-amyloidosis and neurodegeneration among people with normal cognitive function aged 50–89 years: a cross-sectional study. *Lancet Neurology* 2014; 13:997–1005; https://doi.org/10.1016/S1474-4422(14)70194-2 (public access version available at www.ncbi.nlm.nih.gov/pmc/articles/PMC4324499).

2   La Joie R, Visani AV, Baker SL, *et al*. Prospective longitudinal atrophy in Alzheimer's disease correlates with the intensity and topography of baseline tau-PET. *Science Translational Medicine* 2020; eaau5732; https://doi.org/10.1126/scitranslmed.aau5732 (public access version available at www.ncbi.nlm.nih.gov/pmc/articles/PMC7035952).

3   Sevigny J, Chiao P, Bussière T, *et al*. The antibody aducanumab reduces Aβ plaques in Alzheimer's disease. *Nature* 2016; 537:50–56; https://doi.org/10.1038/nature19323.

13 WHEN ARIA IS MORE THAN AN OPERATIC SOLO

Lois and I joked occasionally about my faltering memory when I'd read some riveting novel and chat about it in great detail with her over dinner, then have a hard time remembering it a week later. But one day I woke up unable to read simple words without spelling them out, and there was nothing amusing about it. We were stunned. Everything had been going so well.

Two months earlier, at the end of September 2017, I had the first monthly infusion of the extended trial. Now I knew I was getting aducanu-mab, and had been pleased that for the next month I had no side effects. During the next infusion a month later, the only noticeable side effect was that I experienced a new phantosmia, the illusory smell experiences I'd had occasionally for the past ten years. This one smelled like orange-scented soap and lasted about thirty minutes. It was probably just a coincidence, but I found it encouraging. Maybe it meant the drug was actually going to do something. And then it did.

About a week after the third infusion, the headaches began. They'd last from a few hours to several days. I wasn't particularly concerned because the headaches were very similar to my typical occasional migraines, only more frequent and more severe. But then on December 13, about six weeks into this treatment period, I started having trouble reading simple words. I had to stop and spell them out. It wasn't a dramatic moment when everything written turned to alphabet soup – it was more insidious. The trouble reading was intermittent and sneaked up on me. But it got more frequent and more severe over several days. This was alarming because reading is a major activity for me. I usually read about 100 books a year, as well as keeping up with medical journals and newspapers. Within a week, I couldn't do my crosswords – they might as well have been Rubik's Cubes. Initially, the problem would come and go, and I tried to adapt. Lois suggested I switch to audio books, so I tried one of hers and discovered that I had no trouble understanding spoken language, only written words. My thought at the time was that the difficulty reading was probably a symptom of progression of my Alzheimer's disease. I had the disturbing feeling that this might be my new life: unable to read, unable to drive, unable to do simple calculations.

I call it "my" Alzheimer's disease, and of course the pathology is in my brain alone. I'm also entitled to ownership of the disturbing feeling that this might be "my" new life, that these were "my" problems, "my" frustrations and "my" fears. But, in truth, what happens to me and my life happens to Lois, too. It happens to the family, even with grown kids. I'm sure Lois and the kids were worried, but I'm afraid that one thing Alzheimer's seems to do is impair one's sense of empathy, the ability to understand what others are feeling. There's been a scattering of articles on the connection between decreased empathy and neurodegeneration – nothing comprehensive, but it seems true for me. I haven't lost all capacity for empathy, though. I know because I still try to minimize when these things happen; I don't want to worry Lois. I also am aware that she isn't fooled and she worries any-way. None of that is lost on me. When the diagnosis came through, we did the responsible thing and arranged for legal considerations that will be needed when things get worse. Otherwise, we avoid talking about my day-to-day cognitive scorecard and our respective worries. But this experience of rather marked and sudden cognitive decline was a stark warning of what the future had in store for me – for us. It was unnerving, that sense of certainty about what lay ahead. The only uncertainty was how long it would take to arrive.

About a week later, late one evening, my headache suddenly exploded with excruciating pain. I'd never had a headache this bad. I took my blood pressure and it was alarmingly high, greater than 210/110. I took it several more times thinking I had made an error, but it didn't go down. I was definitely concerned – not freaking out, but very worried. I was pretty sure that something bad was happening.

Afraid I might be having a stroke, I found Lois still up reading and asked her to take me to the hospital. She tends to be very calm in emergencies, which was fortunate because I was quickly crumbling. By the time we arrived, I was confused and couldn't give a coherent history. I was admitted to the intensive care unit (ICU) for IV control of my severe hypertension. A stroke was suspected, but an MRI scan showed that this was not a stroke. There were, however, many areas of brain swelling and microhemorrhages, especially in the left frontal lobe and both temporal lobes. These were the classic imaging findings of ARIA – the areas of bleeding and swelling in the brain – although more extensive and severe than anything previously reported in the neurological literature.

As the night wore on, I remained confused and flummoxed by the simplest cognitive screenings the nurses were giving me every few hours. I was unable to name simple objects like a feather and cactus. It was not looking good. I telephoned my neurologist in San Francisco and left a voice mail to please call me, but I couldn't remember my cell-phone number or how to find it. Fortunately, he returned the call and was able to contact the study doctors and coordinate my care with the ICU staff in Portland.

At some point, I stabilized enough that Lois felt she could leave for a few hours, and for the next few days she came

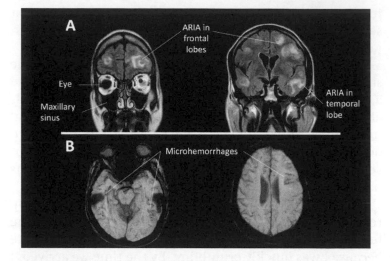

Figure A – These are vertical (imaging) slices through my brain. The white areas are caused by brain swelling in the frontal and temporal lobes. B – These horizontal slices through the brain are optimized to show the iron in blood as black, and they demonstrate multiple tiny black spots of bleeding (microhemorrhages) in both temporal lobes and the left frontal lobe. Small dots of residual iron pigment called hemosiderin are still visible on my most recent MRIs and will probably stay with me for the rest of my life: the tattoo on my brain.

and went, alternating between the ICU and home, where she was cooking ahead for the long-planned holiday dinner we were hosting for our large extended family. While at the hospital, we just kept our eyes on the blood pressure machine, watching and hoping for improvements. Over the next two days, my blood pressure came under control, my confusion improved, and my headache resolved. But I still had trouble reading. Although I could write, I had almost no ability to read even simple words – even when I had just written them myself. I couldn't distinguish between the letters p, b and d. This led to a few amusing text messages that I sent to my son. I was unable to read what I had typed, and the autocorrect took over.

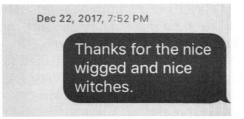

Dec 22, 2017, 7:52 PM

Thanks for the nice wigged and nice witches.

This is a text message that I sent to my son from the ICU during my ARIA episode. I couldn't read what I had typed so the autocorrect did its best. To this day, none of us knows what I was trying to say.

Lois was not amused. However calm, she was clearly concerned. There was no way to know whether this reading problem was permanent, and that possibility hung heavy in the air. It's one thing for me to switch my Goodreads habit from print books to audio books. But there's no simple alternative for so many other ways we all read our way through a day: driving or taking mass transit, reading street signs or simple directions or instructions. Emailing, texting. Telling one pill bottle from another. If I couldn't read, I couldn't safely navigate these ordinary activities alone.

Otherwise much improved and feeling better, I was discharged on Christmas Eve. The city was in the grip of an unexpected snow storm and the home front was a frenzy, but it was such a relief to feel better, I felt euphoric. Lois encouraged me to take it easy; I waved her off. I felt fine! My headache was gone and my reading was a bit better. And I was pumped to prove it and make myself useful. In retrospect, some of that euphoria was probably due to persistent encephalopathy – my brain still wasn't working right. I couldn't hear properly in the lively family conversation around the table, would miss words and then be unable to piece together a full comment from context, as most of us do most of the time without even thinking about it.

In the days ahead, I still required three anti-hypertensive medications to keep my blood pressure down, and I discovered that I could no longer figure a tip when eating out or balance the checkbook, which had never been a problem for me before. It was as if I'd fast-forwarded into a patchy preview of a later-stage Alzheimer's when cognitive function is more seriously impaired. Over the next few weeks, my trouble reading worsened. A repeat MRI scan after a month showed that the brain swelling was actually a little worse despite not getting any more infusions of the test drug. This relapse should not have been surprising since the half-life of aducanumab is about three weeks, meaning it would take fifteen weeks – almost four months – for the drug to be completely eliminated from my blood, and possibly even longer from my brain.

At the time, there were no published recommendations for treatment of severe ARIA like mine. Virtually all cases previously had resolved spontaneously leaving no residual damage to the brain. No one required treatment. My case was considered unique and concerning. You don't have to be a neurologist to know that, as a patient, you never want the words "unique" and "concerning" mentioned together in regard to you and your brain. Several experts in brain swelling and inflammation were consulted, and my doctors decided to treat it as they would a serious flare-up of multiple sclerosis (MS). I didn't have MS, but the inflammatory attacks of MS in the brain share some characteristics of ARIA. I was given five daily infusions of very high-dose steroids. After the third day, my headaches went away and I was able to read again. I had MRI scans every month for the next six months and slowly the areas of brain swelling completely resolved. The only residual MRI abnormalities – the ARIAs – were the tiny spots of iron where the microhemorrhages had been. The blood was gone, but the residual iron pigment called hemosiderin will probably stay with me forever like a tattoo on my brain.

Things got better. Despite some complications as my doctors sorted out the ARIA episode, other side effects of medication, and the neurological twists of Alzheimer's itself, there was steady improvement over the next few months. By the summer of 2018, I was feeling really good. I didn't have headaches and my blood pressure was controlled on the same dose of medication I had taken prior to the ARIA episode. I was back reading my usual six to eight books a month. I could balance the check book on the first try, a task that had been impossible during my ARIA episode, and I began to feel that my memory was actually better than it had been a year – or even two – before. Several factors probably contributed to that, including the addition of a commonly prescribed medication used to treat the symptoms of Alzheimer's. I had started taking donepezil (Aricept) a few months before. Donepezil can cause modest improvement in cognition in people with mild to moderate Alzheimer's disease, and I realized that my sense of improved memory was most likely due, at least in part, to the new medication. But it got me thinking – was it possible that something about that extreme ARIA might have been beneficial? Perhaps there was an unexpected benefit, something new for researchers to explore.

It's hard to imagine how something that objectively bad might actually be beneficial, but the hypothesis isn't as crazy at it might seem. In addition to the abnormal amyloid found in Alzheimer's plaques, amyloid is also found in the walls of small arteries – the vascular system – in the brains of nearly all people with Alzheimer's disease. This vascular amyloid weakens the arteries and can lead to serious bleeding in the brain. It is the most common cause of brain hemorrhages occurring in the elderly in the peripheral parts of the brain [1], in contrast to hypertension, which is the main cause of bleeding occurring deep in the brain.

One possible explanation of why ARIA occur is that medications like the one I was taking – the anti-amyloid monoclonal antibodies, like aducanumab – attack not only the beta-amyloid in plaques within the brain but also the beta-amyloid in the walls of small arteries and capillaries, making these blood vessels leakier. When fluid (plasma) leaks from the blood into the brain, it causes swelling, or edema, there. If red blood cells leak out, they result in microhemorrhages. Both of these are the hallmarks of ARIA on MRI scans.

The protective blood–brain barrier is designed to keep any breaches like that from happening, to keep dangerous pathogens in our blood from circulating directly to the brain. Unlike blood vessels elsewhere in the body, the walls of small arteries and capillaries within the brain have tight, structural barriers that limit the size of molecules that can diffuse from the blood into the fluid bathing the brain. Very small molecules like oxygen and carbon dioxide, as well as sodium and potassium ions, can pass freely across the blood–brain barrier. Some nutrients, like glucose, are actively transported across the blood–brain barrier, but most large molecules such as antibodies, as well as bacteria, viruses and toxins, are usually blocked from entering the brain.

So how can a very large protein like a monoclonal antibody that is purposely infused into the blood ever get into the brain to do the work it's intended to do? The answer is, only a very small fraction of the antibodies cross this blood–brain barrier, unless the barrier is breached – normally an adverse event, since it's designed the way it is to keep the typically larger pathogenic molecules out. This appears to be what is happening in ARIA. Not only can fluid from the blood, and sometimes blood cells as well, leak into the brain, but also the large molecules that are usually blocked by the blood–brain barrier are now able to enter the brain – large molecules like anti-amyloid monoclonal antibodies. An interesting study supports this hypothesis. Researchers analyzed biomarkers for brain amyloid in the

Phase 3 trials of bapineuzu-mab, a monoclonal antibody similar to aducanu-mab, and found that subjects who had received the drug and developed ARIA had greater reduction of beta-amyloid in their brains than those without ARIA [2]. It has even been suggested that ARIA may be a sign of successful engagement of anti-amyloid monoclonal antibodies with beta-amyloid in the brain, and that maybe instead of trying to avoid ARIA in these trials, we should consider using them to improve the effectiveness of these drugs [3].

The blood–brain barrier is in so many ways our species' saving biological grace – nature's essential protective shield. However, that barrier may also hold the key to delivering disease-fighting drugs or other agents directly to the brain to battle disease there, including neurodegenerative diseases like Alzheimer's. Maybe, someday, technology could be used to get monoclonal antibodies through the blood–brain barrier. Although there may well end up being unintended consequences, like toxicity.

My adverse reaction in this clinical trial was no moment of epiphany for Alzheimer's research. I am, as I have noted before, merely anecdotal as far as scientific research is concerned. But my interest in participating in these trials is to contribute what I can – I have no expectations that my involvement in one study or another will permanently change the course of my Alzheimer's. But, although an anecdotal clinical detail can't shape a study, notes are made and discussions are had among clinicians and research scientists, and you never know what anecdotal detail, or accumulation of them, will spark a new idea that leads to a new and productive line of scientific inquiry. To this end, a case study of my ARIA adventure has recently been published in the journal *Alzheimer's & Dementia: Diagnosis, Assessment & Disease Monitoring* [4]. My hope is that some neuroscientist reading that paper will have an "ah ha" moment and think of a new hypothesis to explore. What I am trying to do is to help increase the body of knowledge about how Alzheimer's works, what the mechanisms are that cause loss of brain cells and loss of memory and thinking, and how future treatments might better address the possibility of an effective, disease-modifying treatment.

The fact that I have no illusions that I will directly benefit from any of these trials isn't remarkable – I'm a scientist and that's just how I think. For me, what's exciting is the opportunity to contribute to research as a volunteer participant, for a change, instead of as the clinician, or as the research scientist I'd been so many years earlier. That gave me a sense of purpose and still does. I recognize that the chance of me personally benefiting from a study, in terms of prolonging my life or slowing progression of my Alzheimer's, is very small. What I hope is that my participation will benefit the next generation, my children's generation, so that Alzheimer's becomes a controllable disease within their lifetime, if not within mine. From a personal point of view, it's for my children. That's how I put a face on it. They're at increased risk and I would do anything to help find something to help so it's not an issue for them when they get older. No breakthrough. No magic bullet. But perhaps a block in that pyramid.

And the tattoo on my brain? That tattoo is both literal and figurative. The hemosiderin in my brain is very similar to pigments in the ink used in tattoos. I really do have a tattoo on my brain. Not that anyone's going to see it and admire the artistry. But, hidden though it is, I know it's there, a mark of my battle with Alzheimer's and what came to be a turning point in it for me. Since the earliest days of our kind, a tattoo has always been a signifier, an unashamed assertion of identity or purpose, a mark of belonging to someone or something or some place. Mine is too – a symbol of resistance to the silence that has muted the conversation about Alzheimer's among patients and doctors, family members, and as a society. A reminder to rally attention to help break down the stigma and encourage the important discussions needed to improve the care of those with the disease and to advance the search for a cure.

Chapter-references

1 Viswanathan A, Greenberg SM. Cerebral amyloid angiopathy in the elderly. *Annals of Neurology* 2011; 70:871–880 (public access version available at www.ncbi.nlm.nih.gov/pmc/articles/PMC4004372).

2 Liu E, Wang D, Sperling R, *et al.* Biomarker pattern of ARIA-E participants in phase 3 randomized clinical trials with bapineuzumab. *Neurology* 2018; 90:e877–e886; https://doi.org/10.1212/WNL.0000000000005060.

3 Knopman D.S. Sifting through a failed Alzheimer trial: what biomarkers tell us about what happened. *Neurology* 2018; 90:447–448; https://doi.org/10.1212/WNL.0000000000005073.

4 VandeVrede L, Gibbs DM, Koestler M, *et al.* Symptomatic amyloid-related imaging abnormalities in an ApoE-ε4/ε4 patient treated with aducanumab. *Alzheimer's & Dementia: Diagnosis, Assessment & Disease Monitoring* 2020; 12:e12101; https://doi.org/10.1002/dad2.12101 (open access).

14 MY EXPERIENTIAL LIFE: LIVING WITH EARLY-STAGE ALZHEIMER'S DISEASE

The grilled chicken chunks on Lois's plate glisten with the olive oil, herbs and spices we always use to marinate them before we set the skewers on the grill. Juicy chunks of red pepper, green pepper and onion punctuate the spaces between the tastefully charred chicken bites. Nestled in a bed of brown rice, the whole thing looks like she just lifted her plate from the cover of *Bon Appétit* magazine. Mine, not so much. We are on Day Two of the two-day pre-test elimination diet for an Alzheimer-related clinical trial. More accurately, I am. Researchers are testing an ancient medicinal herb to see how long a specific dose of this extract lasts in my system. In animal studies, a very concentrated tea they've made from this plant produces cognitive improvement in a mouse model of Alzheimer's disease. They hope it will have that effect in humans. I'm their man – or one of eight or so participants in this study.

For them to get a clean reading, they have to be sure that they're starting with a clean slate – that any traces of improvements or healthy components in my blood and urine cannot have been caused by anything else. The anything else includes most of the fresh, healthful foods Lois and I routinely eat, and the olive oil, herbs and spices we use to flavor them. Lois, always the good sport, is having some fun with the concept of the study and has agreed to keep me company on this diet, but in her parallel universe where she gets to eat all the good stuff. We call mine The Unhealthy Diet. No fruits, vegetables, herbs, spices, pepper or flavorings of any kind. No chocolate, coffee, tea or any of the indulgences that have been found to contain some possible health benefits. Also, no ice cream or anything containing vanilla, because something about the vanilla bean can throw things off. This doesn't mean that the approved menu is completely without appeal. Chicken is on the list, although without seasoning. Macaroni and processed cheese, without our usual onion and pepper, is too. Highly processed foods like white bread, Rice Krispies, and white rice get a thumbs-up. Butter is allowed. So are croissants – usually my rare, guilty pleasure. The clinical trial is two days prep, followed by a fasting day down at the hospital for blood draws and urinalyses before, and at multiple intervals after, chugging down about a pint of this very thick but not bad-tasting concoction. Two weeks from now, we'll repeat the prep and tests after a different dose of the brew.

I'm okay eating bland, nutritionally barren foods for two brief periods in the name of science. These small, incremental steps are essential to all scientific advances. By incremental, I mean that this study is strictly about dosage – how much is needed to achieve a consistent measurable presence after it enters your system. This phase of the study is not designed to study the actual effect of that substance on the brain or any of the factors that might relate to developing Alzheimer's. That's for another phase of the study, and it all depends on how precisely scientists are able to determine these matters of dose. I will say this: For the second round of this study, I am going to eat more croissants.

Most of the conversation about Alzheimer's is about fear and loss and things you can't – or eventually won't be able to – do, or do anything about. Helplessness and hopelessness have been the dominant theme of the conversation for more than a century, since Alzheimer's was first identified. It was that way through most of my career because, by the time patients saw their physician with troubling symptoms and were referred on to me for a full neurological work-up, they were already at the moderate or advanced stage of the disease.

It was only in the last five to ten years of my clinical practice, before I retired in 2013, that a few patients were referred to me with the mild cognitive impairment of early-stage dementia. Even then, there wasn't much scientific evidence about lifestyle choices that could slow the progression of Alzheimer's. And for patients diagnosed at those later stages, as were most, the deterioration in the brain was too far advanced to benefit from most of these choices that could have been effective earlier. As a neurologist, I felt utterly helpless being unable to slow down the inexorable march of this disease.

Now, with early-stage Alzheimer's myself, I'm still frustrated that reliably effective medical treatment remains elusive. But I no longer feel helpless to slow down the disease. Along with some medications that may eventually prove beneficial, extensive research now offers strong evidence that certain lifestyle choices about what you eat and what you do each day can benefit the brain and, in some cases, slow the progression of Alzheimer's. But they actually do more than that. So much about Alzheimer's throws you into uncertainty, wipes out assumptions you might have had about yourself, your mind, your capabilities, your future. These fairly simple choices become an organized counterattack against Alzheimer's. As mindful choices, mindful acts, they help provide structure to my thoughts and actions, hope for the future, and a greater sense of happiness and well-being that feels realistic, not merely optimistic. Taking charge, having a sense of being at least to some degree in control, can be an antidote to hopelessness and depression.

As close to a prescription as you can get, the five main anti-Alzheimer's strategies are: (1) aerobic exercise; (2) a Mediterranean-style, or the MIND, diet; (3) mentally stimulating activity; (4) social engagement; and (5) good sleep, along with good control of diabetes, hypertension, high cholesterol, and smoking cessation. Admittedly, these have become such familiar recommendations for a generally healthy lifestyle that they are practically a cliché. It would be easy to shrug them off and put them off for a later time. But for someone with Alzheimer's, or with a strong genetic risk for it, "later" is a gamble. Sooner is the better bet. These strategies have been shown to be most effective in slowing the disease process in the early stages of cell-level changes – the ten to twenty years before significant cognitive impairment. Especially for someone with early-stage Alzheimer's or a significant risk of developing Alzheimer's, this is vital time in your favor. It has been for me.

Once I suspected that I might have Alzheimer's, I set about adopting all five of these recommendations. If my involvement in clinical trials has been my experimental life, then this do-it-yourself regimen has become my experiential life. I've experienced a range of meaningful benefits. Some, like blood pressure and cognitive measures, show in data collected for clinical trials through monitoring devices or real-time cognitive evaluations. Others I've simply recorded in my own case notes. I want to track each of these, and – especially if the effect is positive – I want to stay on that track. My experience is merely my experience – it's personal, anecdotal, not scientific proof of anything. But it doesn't need to be. Rigorous science already provides that.

Consider exercise, for example. If there were a drug for Alzheimer's disease that would slow progression by 50 percent, we'd hail it as a miracle, and it would be worth billions of dollars to the pharmaceutical industry. We already have it, and it is free: exercise. Aerobic exercise has been shown, without a doubt, to have a positive, protective effect, at least in the early stages of the disease. A number of research studies have shown up to 50 percent decline in the rate of developing Alzheimer's among those who start the study with no clinical evidence of dementia [1]. In virtually all studies on people with early-stage disease including mild cognitive impairment, there appears to be unequivocal benefit, not only in slowing cognitive decline, but specifically in reducing the rate of brain shrinkage related to amyloid [2]. In addition to these long-term benefits of exercise in slowing cognitive decline, there is also evidence for a modest and transitory acute effect of exercise – meaning that your brain is sharper during exercise than when not exercising [3]. Mine is, and reliably so. I am most able to think clearly and creatively during, and for a few hours after, exercising, even if it is just walking the dog. Some of this may be due to fewer distractions, but the noticeable boost of cognitive function is real for me. In those moments, I can feel the stepped-up cognitive traction as I read, write, listen, think or talk with others.

Even modest levels of exercise are helpful, but there does seem to be a dose–response effect: more activity is more effective than less activity. Also, the sooner the exercise regimen is started, the more positive effect it will likely have. In the later stages of dementia, exercise may improve mobility, but it doesn't seem to improve cognition [4]. For those with early-stage disease, those with a family history or those with known positive APOE-4 carrier status, it is especially important to start a regular exercise program. Starting it at earlier ages, in the forties if possible, is better than waiting until the sixties or seventies. One recent study suggests that the benefit of exercise is not as robust in those who carry the APOE-4 gene [5], and it may be even more important for those people to start their exercise regimen as early as possible. The optimal amount of exercise is not yet clear. I aim for at least 10,000 steps a day, but recent research has found that 8,000 steps or even fewer may be beneficial.

Other encouraging findings specific to Alzheimer's disease support each of the recommended brain-healthy lifestyle choices around diet, stimulating mental activity, social interaction and sleep.

The data for a beneficial effect of diet is strong, if not quite as robust yet as that for exercise. Most studies have shown that a Mediterranean-style diet promotes brain health, as well as cardiovascular health. A modification of the Mediterranean diet called the DASH diet (Dietary Approaches to Stop Hypertension) was designed with the goal of lowering high blood pressure, and it too had a modest effect on slowing cognitive decline with aging. In 2015, the MIND diet (Mediterranean–DASH Intervention for Neurodegenerative Delay) was introduced to specifically target slowing of cognitive deterioration, both in normal aging and in Alzheimer's disease. The MIND diet combines most elements of the Mediterranean and DASH diets, but specifically focuses on foods that have the most evidence for benefits to brain health, such as whole grains, green-leafy vegetables, beans, nuts and berries. One study followed 923 community residents 58–98 years of age, who did not have Alzheimer's at onset, for an average of 4½ years on the MIND diet. Those who stuck to the diet even moderately developed Alzheimer's disease at a 35 percent lower rate than those with poor adherence to the diet. Those with high adherence to the diet did even better, developing Alzheimer's at a 53 percent lower rate than those with poor adherence [6]. It thus appears that just a good effort at following the diet can lower the risk of developing Alzheimer's. (See more about the MIND diet, recommended foods and servings in the Appendix.)

The number of studies on the effect of diet in moderating risk for Alzheimer's lags a bit behind that for exercise. But they are coming. A recent study in the journal *Neurology* concluded that higher dietary intakes of flavonols – found in citrus, berries, apples, legumes and red wine – may be associated with reduced risk of developing Alzheimer's dementia [7]. Most studies of the Mediterranean and DASH diets tend to show a benefit for brain health, but the MIND diet appears to be the most effective [8]. Hopefully, additional studies will confirm these findings. If so, the benefit of diet may rival that of exercise.

Personally, I am operating on that assumption. I've adopted the MIND diet along with my exercise regimen. Comparing the two from a purely personal perspective, I can feel the cognitive boost during and after exercise, and the real-time data from my tracking devices confirms that. I can't say that I feel a noticeable boost after eating an avocado or a bowl of nuts and berries. But I do know that all together, and eaten as a steady diet, these food choices have been proven to be beneficial in other ways that are factors in the development of – or protection against – Alzheimer's. That's good enough for me.

Admittedly, it wasn't a sharp turn from my eating habits all along, and there's so much variety and flexibility, it's not as if it I've suffered a sacrifice on my plate. Most nights, I'm in charge of the salad, Lois the main dish, and she's a great cook. My only disappointment has nothing to do with the food choices. It's the fact that my senses of smell and taste have been hijacked by Alzheimer's, so I miss the aromas and flavors that were always like a sensory appetizer before Lois served up her latest creation. Now Jack's the one with the early-warning for aromatics.

Moving from meals to the mind, participating in mentally stimulating activity has long been shown to postpone the onset of cognitive impairment caused by Alzheimer's disease. As early as 2001, a group from Rush Medical School began looking at the effects of various types of leisure activity on the chance of later developing dementia. Intellectual activities (reading, playing games or going to classes) and social activities (visiting or being visited by friends or relatives, going out to movies or restaurants or clubs or centers, doing voluntary community work, and attending religious services) all significantly delayed the onset of dementia. The authors proposed that "maintaining intellectual and social engagement through participation in everyday activities seems to buffer healthy individuals against cognitive decline in later life" [9]. More recent studies have generally confirmed this. Activities pursued in late life – such as reading books five to seven days a week, using a computer three to seven days a week, participating in social activities two to four days a week, and doing craft activities – all lead to about a 30 percent reduction in the rate of developing cognitive impairment. Those who do these activities in both middle and late life have even greater benefit, and the benefit increases with the number of these activities done, to a maximum of about a 50 percent reduction in the rate of developing cognitive impairment [10].

I'm personally convinced of the importance of mental stimulation in slowing the progression of cognitive impairment. My experience, anecdotal though it is, informs my thinking on the science that may underlie it. Although I don't have evidence to support it, my theory is that mental stimulation helps to develop alternate circuits in the brain so that, as Alzheimer's progresses and some neural pathways fail, there can be backup pathways to help out. This may be just another way of saying that it builds cognitive reserve.

I make a determined effort to keep my brain active – engaged, and often challenged – as much of the time as possible. I read books every day, on average two or three per week. I read a mix of fiction and nonfiction. I'm having increasing trouble remembering what I have read a few days later, so I tell Lois about what I have been reading to help firm up those memories. She has been a supremely good sport about it. Keeping track of my reading on the Goodreads webpage has also been helpful.[1] Even though I may not remember much about a book a week or two after reading it, I still enjoy it in the moment.

I have been keeping a journal since I first started losing my sense of smell fourteen years ago. Not only does my journal provide a record of facts about my medical history I might have forgotten, but the act of writing helps me organize and consolidate my memory of events. Except for the time that I was affected by ARIA, my ability to do calculations has remained good. I still balance the checkbook and often get it right the first time. As a mental exercise, I try to do multiplication and division problems in my head, but that is getting much harder as I can no longer remember carry-over numbers and other intermediate steps long enough to complete the calculation. I play the piano for fun. It has been suggested to me that learning new pieces on an instrument is more stimulating to the brain than simply playing old favorites, so I do both, struggling through new pieces, and then rewarding myself with a familiar piece that my fingers still remember how to play. This fits the neurological schematic in that procedural memory, the automatic memory of how to do things like ride a bike or play an instrument, is located deep in the brain in the basal ganglia and cerebellum and is preserved much longer in Alzheimer's disease than the declarative

---

[1]   I have been using Goodreads since 2008. It allows me to get ideas for books to read and to keep lists of books to read in the future, as well as of books I have already read. I find it to be very useful and refer to it multiple times a day. One word of caution: Goodreads was bought by Amazon a few years ago, so expect to get suggestions about books in which you might be interested. I don't find this to be intrusive, but some might: www.goodreads.com.

memory for words and numbers located primarily in the temporal lobes. I limit passive activities like watching TV to only thirty to sixty minutes of news per day and an occasional sporting event.

Social engagement is also important, and it can be hard in Alzheimer's disease. Apathy is almost universal, especially in the later stages. I've never been especially social. I don't particularly like to go to parties – now more than ever. Part of this is the trouble I have understanding language when several people are talking at once. It's really difficult for me to follow the conversations in a group, so I tend to stop trying. I also continue to have some trouble recognizing faces, even of people I know fairly well. This prosopagnosia, or face blindness, is usually due to damage to the fusiform gyrus of the temporal lobe or to portions of the occipital lobes. It is relatively common in Alzheimer's, and it is just one more thing that makes social interaction somewhat fraught. Having said that, I realize that one way to fight the apathy is to stay socially engaged and not withdraw into a protective shell, so I do make an effort. I spend a lot of time with my three children and four grandchildren. I chat with neighbors while working in the front yard or walking Jack. I see old friends regularly, and I stay in touch with my neurology colleagues at OHSU and around the world.

Sleep research brings insights literally from bench to bedside. Sleep apnea can cause cognitive impairment that may mimic or worsen impairment due to Alzheimer's, and it should be ruled out or treated if present. Other sleep disturbances are common in Alzheimer's disease, especially in the moderate and late stages. It often is difficult for the patient with Alzheimer's to get adequate sleep. However, it is becoming increasingly clear that adequate sleep may be very important in fighting the accumulation of amyloid in the brain, at least in the early stages of the disease. There is evidence from both mouse and human studies that amyloid is scavenged from the brain during sleep. This is thought to occur through the so-called glymphatic circulation in the brain, a network of passages that surround brain blood vessels and bathe the brain in fluid. The glymphatic system gets its name because of the similarity to the lymphatic vessels that are seen throughout the rest of the body [11]. During the non-REM, slow-wave stage of sleep in humans, waves of fluid pulse through the glymphatic passages in the brain, and these fluid waves are driven by both arterial pulsations and changes in the electrical activity of the brain [12]. This washing of the brain during slow-wave sleep appears to remove toxins, including beta-amyloid. Reports of this research in the popular press have led to the inevitable headlines about "brainwashing." This is still a new, but very exciting, field of study. There are hopes that methods might be found for manipulating this system to enhance amyloid removal. This is years off, but, in the meantime, I make a point of getting at least seven and a half hours of sleep per night.

For those with diabetes or hypertension, it is especially important to get these well controlled as soon as possible. There are probably several ways that these conditions increase risk of dementia, either by directly facilitating Alzheimer's pathology or by causing microvascular damage in the brain that leads to multiple tiny strokes. Recall that the brains of many patients who clinically appear to have Alzheimer's disease have not only amyloid plaques and neurofibrillary tangles when examined after death – the pathological hallmarks of Alzheimer's disease – but also evidence of mini-strokes that can result in vascular dementia. The high blood glucose levels and insulin resistance in tissues throughout the body, including the brain, in type 2 diabetes appear to promote propagation of both amyloid and tau pathology in the brain [13].

All of these lifestyle changes that appear to be beneficial in slowing the progression of amyloid accumulation and onset of cognitive impairment share one important caveat: they work best in the earliest stages of the disease, probably in the period when amyloid has started to accumulate but before significant cognitive impairment has started. The pre-symptomatic period of Alzheimer's disease that can last ten or even twenty years is a critical time, then, for meaningful intervention. By the time Alzheimer's has reached the moderate and late stages, many nerve cells have been destroyed, and we don't have a clue yet how to make them regenerate. No lifestyle modification is likely to have much of an effect at this stage, above increasing comfort and well-being. A large study from the UK on exercise in patients with moderate-stage dementia showed no benefit [14]. It's too late. And this was exactly the time in the course of the disease that we were making the diagnosis twenty and thirty years ago. It was too late then, and it is still too late now.

It is also very likely that the first effective, disease-modifying drugs, drugs that will slow progression of Alzheimer's or even lead to a cure, will work best in these earliest stages of the disease – again, before any cognitive symptoms have occurred.

It has been more than 100 years since Auguste's diagnosis, and death five years later. Yet, until fairly recently, the typical time from diagnosis to death for both early- and late-onset Alzheimer's disease has remained the same: about eight years. What's wrong with this picture? When we know, as we do now, that the earliest changes in the brain associated with later Alzheimer's disease start at least ten if not twenty years before any cognitive symptoms are noticed, how can we ignore that window of opportunity for intervention?

Some argue that that there's no need to make an early diagnosis – just encourage everyone to adopt these lifestyle changes as early as possible to lessen their chances of getting Alzheimer's in late life. That seems reasonable, and I'm sure that some people might do that. But most of us, when we are in our thirties, forties and fifties, are incredibly busy with family, careers and our hopes and dreams. There may not be much bandwidth left – neither time nor energy – to concentrate on preventing a hypothetical disaster far in the future. I can tell you that there was nothing like the jolt of finding that I was APOE-4 positive, and that I had amyloid in my brain, to get my attention and motivate me to start doing everything I could to learn how I could mitigate the almost certain prospect of Alzheimer's.

In the years since, the link between lifestyle choices and genetic predisposition has become only more compelling. Rudoph Tanzi is a pioneering researcher in the genetics of Alzheimer's disease who is recognized for his discovery of three rare genes that result in autosomal-dominant, hereditary Alzheimer's disease, as well as many other genes that appear to increase risk without always causing the disease. Dr. Tanzi has described how the expression of these risk genes – the epigenetics – can be altered by our lifestyle.

"Every choice we make leads to experiences that change the expression of our genes," Tanzi told the US Senate Special Committee on Aging in 2019 [15].

> Gene expression is actually controlled by our habits. A healthy lifestyle of good habits leads to beneficial gene programs and good health. The opposite is also true. You may currently have bad habits, like a little too much junk food, which induce gene expression programs that promote risk for age-related disease. But, with repetition, the establishment of new, "good habits," like a plant-rich diet, will change gene expression programs that promote health … At the end of the day, by altering our gene expression programs through our daily conscious choices, we have the power to slow the aging process, improve mood, staving off anxiety and depression, reduce persistent aches and pains, improve quality of sleep, and even decrease risk of age-related chronic diseases including cancer and neurodegenerative diseases.

Tanzi emphasized that the benefits of these simple lifestyle choices hold promise far beyond the roughly six million of us in the USA with Alzheimer's or those at significant risk of it. "It is estimated that another 30 million Americans harbor brain pathology, such as amyloid plaques and tangles, that substantially increases their risk for symptoms of dementia over the next 5 to 15 years. ... While we wait for effective drugs, we must in parallel consider whether we can stave off Alzheimer's via life-style and behavioral interventions." [15]

The best part is that, although these prescriptive lifestyle steps are based on complex science, there's nothing necessarily complicated about doing them. Often they overlap, which I believe may have a synergistic effect, heightening the overall benefit. However you do it, ultimately it all becomes part of your own experiential life. Against the inevitable encroachments of Alzheimer's, I've held my own for this moment, this day, this experience. Not "in spite of Alzheimer's," but, in fact, living with it and exploiting the slower, early-stage aspects of the disease to expand my time to claim this quality of life.

One early morning, I am well into my breakfast and coffee routine, my laptop on the table to check a few things, when Jack trots into the kitchen with a jaunty air and sits at attention by my chair. He announces his presence with the beady-eyed stare he has perfected to serve as my cue to put on my trail shoes and take us both out for our daily walk through Forest Park. Jack makes an eager walking companion in my quest to get at least 10,000 steps per day of aerobic exercise. We walk the trails in the sprawling forest preserve, sometimes enjoying only the company of the native plants and wildlife. When we meet fellow walkers, people and dogs alike, we swap notes from the trail and dog tales. The dogs do their own version of swapping intel.

That morning, we log three miles over an hour and 20 minutes. It goes fast, with just a few breaks for trail encounters, including a man and his dog, whom Jack warms up to once they've had a chance to prove to him that they're no threat. Once we're back at the house, for Jack, it's time for a nap. For me, the exercise has recharged my brain and I'm in optimum mode for reading, writing, following up on phone calls or sitting down at the piano to play some Bach or Chopin. Lois is out. Across the room, her current puzzle is about half finished; it's safe from me. I'm more into crosswords than jigsaw puzzles. This time tomorrow, our kids will bring the four grandkids over for Sunday waffles, reading and playtime with us. Our youngest grandchild is ten months old, the others are two, three and five years old. It promises to be an active day. They'll run me ragged around the house and yard, want to read books and play games, need some coaching through the occasional spat and meltdown, and push a few boundaries. I'm not complaining. All that comes with a good dose of love and laughter – the best medicine.

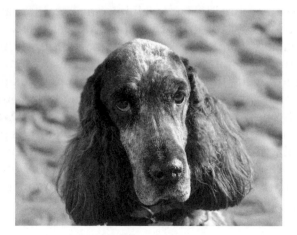

Jack, my walking buddy.

Chapter-references

1 Buchman AS, Boyle PA, Yu L, *et al.* Total daily physical activity and the risk of AD and cognitive decline in older adults. *Neurology* 2012; 78:1323–1329 (public access version available at www.ncbi.nlm.nih.gov/ pmc/articles/PMC3335448).

2 Rabin JS, Klein H, Kirn DR, *et al.* Associations of physical activity and β-amyloid with longitudinal cognition and neurodegeneration in clinically normal older adults. *JAMA Neurology* 2019; 76:1203–1210 (public access version available at www.ncbi.nlm.nih .gov/pmc/articles/PMC6635892).

3 Chang YK, Labban JD, Gapin JI, *et al.* The effects of acute exercise on cognitive performance: a meta-analysis. *Brain Research* 2012; 1453:87–101; https://doi .org/10.1016/j.brainres.2012.02.068.

4 Sanders LMJ, Hortobágyi T, Karssemeijer EGA, *et al.* Effects of low- and high-intensity physical exercise on physical and cognitive function in older persons with dementia: a randomized controlled trial. *Alzheimer's Research & Therapy* 2020; 12:28; https://doi.org/10.1186/ s13195-020-00597-3.

5 Licher S, Ahmad S, Karamujić-Čomić H, *et al.* Genetic predisposition, modifiable-risk-factor profile and long-term dementia risk in the general population. *Nature Medicine* 2019; 25:1364–1369 (public access version available at www.ncbi.nlm.nih.gov/pmc/articles/ PMC6739225).

6 Morris MC, Tangney CC, Wang Y, *et al.* MIND diet associated with reduced incidence of Alzheimer's disease. *Alzheimer's & Dementia* 2015; 11:1007–1014 (public access version available at www.ncbi.nlm.nih .gov/pmc/articles/PMC4532650).

7 Holland TM, Agarwal P, Wang Y, *et al.* Dietary flavanols and risk of Alzheimer dementia. *Neurology*

2020; 94:e1749–e1756 (public access version available at www.ncbi.nlm.nih.gov/pmc/articles/PMC7282875).

8 Hosking DE, Eramudugolla R, Cherbuin N and Anstey KJ. MIND not Mediterranean diet related to 12-year incidence of cognitive impairment in an Australian longitudinal cohort study. *Alzheimer's & Dementia* 2019; 15:581–589; https://doi.org/10.1212/WNL.0000000000008981.

9 Scarmeas N, Levy G, Tang MX, *et al.* Influence of leisure activity on the incidence of Alzheimer's disease. *Neurology* 2001; 57:2236–2242 (public access version available at www.ncbi.nlm.nih.gov/pmc/articles/PMC3025284).

10 Krell-Roesch J, Syrjanen JA, Vassilaki M, *et al.* Quantity and quality of mental activities and the risk of incident mild cognitive impairment. *Neurology* 2019; 93:e548–e558 (open access).

11 Jessen NA, Munk ASF, Lundgaard I, *et al.* The glymphatic system – a beginner's guide. *Neurochemical Research* 2015; 40:2583–2599 (public access version available at www.ncbi.nlm.nih.gov/pmc/articles/PMC4636982).

12 Fultz NE, Bonmassar G, Setsompop K, *et al.* Coupled electrophysical, hemodynamic, and cerebrospinal fluid oscillations in human sleep. *Science* 2019; 366:628–631 (public access version available at www.ncbi.nlm.nih.gov/pmc/articles/PMC7309589).

13 Li X, Song D, Leng SX. Link between type 2 diabetes and Alzheimer's disease: from epidemiology to mechanism and treatment. *Clinical Interventions in Aging* 2015; 10:549–560; https://doi.org/10.2147/CIA.S74042 (public access version available at www.ncbi.nlm.nih.gov/pmc/articles/PMC4360697).

14 Lam SE, Sheehan B, Atherton N, *et al.* Dementia and Physical Activity (DAPA) trial of moderate to high intensity exercise training for people with

dementia: randomised controlled trial. *BMJ* 2018; 361:k1675; https://doi.org/10.1136/bmj.k1675 (open access).

15 Testimony of Dr. Rudolph Tanzi – Promoting healthy aging: living your best life long into your golden years – presented to the US Senate Special Committee on Aging, September 25, 2019; https://www.aging .senate.gov/imo/media/doc/SCA_Tanzi_09_25_19.pdf.

15 MADELEINES, MUSIC AND AFRICAN DOVES

Musing from his sickbed, Marcel Proust in his 1913 semi-autographical novel *Remembrances of Things Past* (*À la recherche du temps perdu*) famously described the vivid retrieval of a long-lost memory evoked by the smell and taste of a tea-soaked madeleine cake. His childhood memory of cherished Sunday mornings in the country, his aunt Léonie, and now the rush of memory itself was an exquisite pleasure, he wrote. "And all from my cup of tea." The Proust effect, as it has come to be called, refers to the phenomenon most of us have experienced, in which sensory cues instantly take us back to a long-ago memory.[1]

Modern science has since established that taste and smell cues are perhaps the strongest stimuli for retrieving old memories. Smell, in particular, can evoke memories from earlier in life than any other type of sensory stimulus. Today, the scientific literature tells the deeper story of the neurological interconnections between smell – the brain's olfactory sense – and memory. It goes far beyond the emotional connection expressed in Proust's madeleine reverie. Neuroscience tells us that, more than a catalyst for remembrances of things past, the olfactory sense and the regions of the brain that process smell, the neurons that carry those messages and the pathways they travel, may be uniquely important in how the brain consolidates different types of memory that help us pay attention, listen

---

[1] For a wide-ranging discussion of sensory memory cues in relation to psychology, literature, art, music, cuisine and aromatherapy, see the book by Cretien van Campen [1].

and discern, reflect and learn, and respond to the world around us [2]. For this reason, the olfactory processing areas in the brain – such as the olfactory bulb, piriform cortex and orbital frontal cortex – have unique aspects of structure and function that also may hold valuable information about how Alzheimer's develops and spreads.

In short, the science suggests that, when the sense of smell goes missing, it can disrupt the mechanism for making and retrieving stored memories; its absence, or dysfunction, is a red flag that something in the architecture of the brain's processing system may be amiss. Like the canary in the coal mine, when the olfactory sense keels over, it's a signal – non-specific, but nonetheless significant – that possible disease-related changes may be under way in the brain.

The relationship between olfactory dysfunction and Alzheimer's disease was described in scientific literature by the 1990s, but it wasn't widely known by physicians, including practicing neurologists like myself, at that time. While the relationship between loss of smell and Parkinson's was more widely recognized, the difference was probably that Alzheimer's patients, by the time they were first seen by a neurologist, were cognitively impaired and unlikely to mention or even recognize smell issues, whereas most Parkinson's patients at the time of their diagnosis were not cognitively impaired. Even when it happened to me – when I first noticed that I couldn't smell the roses back in the summer of 2006 – it didn't occur to me that this might be a harbinger of Alzheimer's disease. I didn't know yet about my heightened genetic risk for Alzheimer's, so it was nowhere on my radar.

Since that time, the connection between olfactory dysfunction and Alzheimer's has become more widely recognized [3]. Loss of smell is now considered a biomarker for Alzheimer's, as newer findings have continued to confirm the connection. In the purely scientific sense, they haven't added much new information to our understanding of the phenomenon. But they are meaningful blocks in the pyramid of scientific advancement.

I don't want to make a big deal out of this singular piece of my own anecdotal case story. To me, olfactory loss is just one more portal into the explorations that, in time, will lead us to substantive ways in which we can spot changes that may predict Alzheimer's and enable us to intervene sooner, or perhaps even prevent Alzheimer's disease.

Lately, with the luxury of time and freedom to reflect more broadly on these sensory aspects of Alzheimer's as I live with them, I am cognizant of what Alzheimer's has taken away, as well as what has been spared – at least for the time being.

As for the sensory losses, they have been slow and incremental, their impact more poignant or practical than painful. I still can't smell roses. The bouquet of a good wine is lost on me. The sigh-worthy smell of Lois's apple pie or roast chicken wafting through the house goes undetected by me, though Jack's move toward the kitchen serves as a trusty visual cue. Smell makes up a large part of what we perceive as taste, so, not surprisingly, food tastes bland to me unless it's highly spiced. (Hot spices are sensed by taste buds and by pain receptors of the trigeminal nerve, so those aspects of taste are intact.) One distinct advantage of my olfactory loss: when there's something smelly to clean up, I'm the go-to guy – and I genuinely don't mind.

Earlier in my life, I never forgot a face. Now I do. Or, more accurately, I don't recognize them out of context. One of the most common visual problems in Alzheimer's is face blindness, or prosopagnosia. Normally, when sensory information gets to the brain, it is processed in a variety of complex ways that create context and meaning. Is that smell similar to another we have experienced? All the sensory information we hear, see, smell, taste and touch is intertwined this way, contextualized in time and space and emotional texture. Like the words we hear or read on the page, it's only when they're strung together in a sentence that they carry meaning for us. Even if one or more of those words is indecipherable, we still tend to glean the meaning from context. Is that face you see someone you know or a stranger? Most of the time, it's an easy call. For many people with Alzheimer's disease, it isn't, once this complex sensory processing system becomes impaired. As mine is.

I can no longer reliably identify a neighbor or other casual acquaintance by just looking at their face. If I can see their car, their dog, or hear them speak, those additional contextual clues make it so that I generally have no trouble identifying them. But often their face alone is no longer enough. Prosopagnosia is usually due to problems with the inferior, posterior portions of the temporal lobes and adjacent occipital lobes. That's how it showed up in my second tau PET scan in 2018 (see Color Plate 2); the abnormal tau protein had spread into this area on both sides of the brain. Other visual problems can occur in Alzheimer's, such as hallucinations, visual distortions and even cortical blindness – partial or total loss of vision – but these are more likely to occur late in the disease.

And you won't find me up on the roof cleaning the gutters out anymore. Proprioception, the awareness of where we are in space, is based on multiple sensory inputs to the brain, including touch receptors, position sensors in our muscles and joints, vision, and input from the vestibular (balance) apparatus in our inner ear. These inputs are integrated in multiple areas of the brain, normally producing an accurate sense of which way is up, balance, and the kind of body awareness that lets your left hand know what the right is doing, literally. Proprioception is often impaired in Alzheimer's, even in the early stages. I've noticed that my balance is not as good as it used to be. So I don't go up on the roof – not a great loss in and of itself. And I always use the handrail when going down stairs, which is frequent in our old two-story home. The stout, creaky staircase we taught our three children to navigate with hands on the rail requires the same of me now. Still, to our young grandchildren just learning to navigate steps themselves, I pass for a doting grandfather modeling safe technique.

A common thread here is that multiple types of complex brain processing of sensory information can be impaired by Alzheimer's, some in the early stages and some later in the disease. A remarkable exception is music. For reasons that are still not fully understood, the abilities to enjoy, identify and even play music are often preserved even into the latest stages of the disease. This is most apparent in those who have been professional musicians, some of whom can play very complicated pieces on their instruments even after they have lost the ability to communicate verbally [4].

While smells can no longer trigger fond memories for me as they did for Proust, my other senses can – music, perhaps, most of all. Even something so simple as a birdsong. On a recent walk with Jack along a path through the shore pines on the Oregon coast, I heard the distinctive, plaintive call of the Eurasian collared dove (*Streptopelia decaocto*) and was immediately transported to Africa, to my friend William Howlett's veranda, where we would watch the sun set on Mt. Kilimanjaro every evening while enjoying a beer after a clinical day at the hospital. The redeyed dove (*Streptopelia semitorquato*) is the most common dove in that part of Tanzania, and its call is so distinctive that it felt like a greeting whenever I arrived each spring to volunteer. The Eurasian collared dove is a fairly recent immigrant to the US. Several escaped from a pet store in the Bahamas in 1974 during an attempted robbery, and by 1980 the species had found its way to Florida. It quickly spread throughout the US, reaching Oregon in 1988. Now, near my home in Portland, I am almost as likely to hear the collared dove as I am to hear the more familiar mourning dove (*Zenaide macroura*). The Eurasian collared dove's call is very similar to its African cousin, and when I first heard it a couple of years ago in Portland I was pleasantly surprised by the rush of good feeling associated with it, undiminished by Alzheimer's.

Music is my madeleine. Music not only calms me, but puts me in touch with my increasingly forgotten past, rich autobiographical memories that place me in time and among people and in places in those formative years that made me *me*. The Beatles' "Michelle" reliably transports me to my bedroom as a teen, listening to the radio, and sighing over unrequited love. If a song I haven't heard for fifty years or more comes on the radio, it immediately tags a memory from the time I used to listen to it. It seems I always have a song going in my head. Not the annoying kind that sticks when you wish it wouldn't, but one you welcome. I take the time to give these reveries their due. Music turns nostalgia into a kind of neurological resistance to a disease that takes no prisoners.

Daniel Levitin, in his illuminating book *This Is Your Brain on Music*, about the brain processes involved in listening to and making music, gives us some clues as to why the functions of the brain involved with music seem to be so resilient to the ravages of Alzheimer's. First off, he notes, "musical activity involves nearly every region of the brain that we know about and nearly every neural subsystem" [5]. When areas of the brain are damaged, nearby areas can sometimes take over the function of the damaged area, in the process called "neuroplasticity." Since the processing of music involves so much of the brain, it might be more likely that there will be one of these nearby areas with similar function that can take over the work of brain areas damaged by Alzheimer's. Interestingly, the rhythm of music is appreciated and produced in the cerebellum and basal ganglia. Both of these brain areas are involved in procedural memory – the type of memory we use to ride a bike or play a piano – and these are the most resistant areas of the brain to the pathology of Alzheimer's. It might seem far-fetched to think that the beat in a Beatles song and the rhythmic coordination required to ride a bike have anything in common, but in the brain's architecture and circuitry, they're wired together.

MRI studies of the brains of professional musicians show some other clues that may help us understand the resilience of our musical brain. Presumably due to many years of daily practice, the brains of these musicians show enlargement in three key areas: (1) the planum temporale located on the superior aspect of the temporal lobe; (2) the primary motor cortex; and (3) the anterior corpus callo-sum, the connecting cable that allows the right and left sides of the brain to communicate [6]. None of these areas is affected by Alzheimer's pathology until late in the dis-ease. All of this suggests that key areas for music appreci-ation and production are spread throughout the brain, and some of the most important areas are in regions that are relatively resistant to attack by Alzheimer's disease.

Not only is music appreciation, identification and pro-duction – the ability to make music – relatively preserved in Alzheimer's, it is becoming increasingly clear that involve-ment in listening to music and making music, whether it be singing or playing an instrument, can help slow cogni-tive decline in Alzheimer's disease and enhance autobio-graphical memory, the memory of events from the past [7].

My mental playlist is heavy on the music I loved in my teens and twenties, songs or even ambient sounds that re-vive memories of good times: playing poker and bridge with friends on Friday nights, playing soccer and running track after school, surfing as often as I could, and playing lead guitar in a school rock band called Tujunga Next Exit. I've probably worn a dedicated neural pathway for "Hotel Cali-fornia," just about my favorite song of all time, but there's no evidence to suggest that music in the brain displaces more important connections, and I doubt it contributes to cognitive impairment. What I can say is that these songs in my head have become even more noticeable in the past few years as I have started to have more cognitive impairment from Alzheimer's. Music may also help to ameliorate neuropsychiatric symptoms such as agitation and depression, common in the later stages of Alzheimer's but not unusual earlier, as I've experienced both. Music therapy is becoming an integral part of the management of Alzheimer's disease. Many memory and aging clinics, as well as local chapters of the Alzheimer's Association, have choirs or other musical activities for people with dementia.

Once a week, Lois takes off with Jack to obedience training class, and that is my cue to sit down at the keyboard. This is my practice time, too, as I work my way through some of the easier Beethoven sonatas that Uncle Fred left to me, along with the Steinway baby grand that he played daily for all of his adult life. Most of these are still beyond my skill level – even before Alzheimer's factored in – but I continue to enjoy the challenge they pose for me. What's more, between the concentration required and the familiar routine of practice lies a simple pleasure where memory and music intersect. The sound of that piano and the trendy Hammond electric organ he eventually acquired became part of the musical backdrop of my childhood from the time I was about ten. Uncle Fred had always worked his way through all of the Beethoven sonatas in order each year, and he continued to do so despite worsening cognitive impairment. He ultimately required placement in a care facility, where he died in 1974 at age 85 from what was almost certainly Alzheimer's disease.

My mother played piano too, and saw to it that I and my two older sisters took lessons and practiced, dutifully if not enthusiastically. My dad and I would hang out with Uncle Fred on Saturdays, and while those two took their coffee and mechanical tinkering to a backyard workbench, I'd either join them or stay in and practice piano. Once through that necessity, time on the Hammond was my reward. I staged my musical insurrection in high school, abandoning piano to play lead guitar in my high school rock band.

I took for granted my mother's gift for the piano – that she would sight-read Beethoven, Bach, and even Rachmaninoff's Prelude in C# minor, a piece I have always loved but have never been able to master myself, let alone sight-read. It finally registered on me how good she was when I was learning the trumpet in college. I came home one weekend with my trumpet, showing off a Bach Air transcribed for trumpet that I really loved. She sat down at the piano and played the very challenging piano accompaniment with me. It was a magical moment as we made music together, possibly, as I realized later, for the first and last time.

I usually wait until Lois and Jack are out the door before I sit down at the piano to play. Despite evidence-based assurances that I'm unlikely to lose these skills, I worry that, if it does happen, Lois will be too kind to say anything about it even as the deterioration adds to her worries.

In my musical brain, which guides my eyes across the page and my fingers across the keys, my eccentric Uncle Fred is in good company with Proust's aunt Léonie, both whisked forward on a neuronic whim – time travelers who exist only in my memory.

However less frequent, some other sensory memories remain vibrant as well. Warm sand on my back is one. It's been a long time since I've felt warm sand on my back – probably more than ten years ago, on our last trip to Hawaii. Warm sand isn't a feature on Oregon's brisk coast, and certainly not in combination with a bare back. But there was something about that sensation on my back when I would lie down in the sand that would take me back to the summers of my youth. Our family had a trailer at the beach near Laguna Beach in Southern California from the time I was eight. My mother and sisters and I spent pretty much the whole summer there each year, and my father would come down on weekends. So I would spend every day at the beach and at the pool, swimming and playing with friends. As I got older I took up surfing. My skin burnt to a crisp, undoubtedly leading to trouble later in life with various skin cancers, including two melanomas, but I felt free and invincible at the time.

Perhaps these sensory triggers of distant memories are even more acute now that I have no sense of smell. That's not something I can measure, but they seem so. Whatever the explanation, most importantly at this moment in time, insights like these tell us that there are many, subtle ways the brain begins to change that make it vulnerable to neurodegenerative disease, long before our current methods for diagnosis are able to detect it. Whatever science is eventually able to explain – or not – it makes for a curious sensory puzzle, this phenomenon of receding capacities alongside resilient ones, even in the context of neurodegenerative processes. Curious and, in some ways, encouraging.

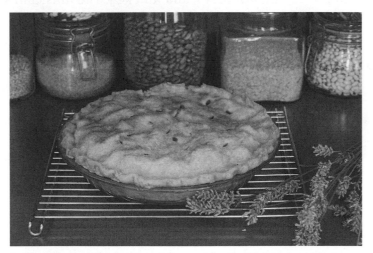

Lois' apple pie. This is one of the aromas that I once loved but can no longer smell.

Chapter-references

1   van Campen C, *The Proust Effect: The Senses as Doorways to Lost Memories*. Oxford University Press, 2014.
2   Andrews-Hanna JR. The brain's default network and its adaptive role in internal mentation. *Neuroscientist* 2012; 18(3):251–270; https://doi.org/10.1177/1073858411403316 (public access version available at www.ncbi.nlm.nih.gov/pmc/articles/PMC3553600).
3   Zou YM, Lu D, Liu LP, *et al.* Olfactory dysfunction in Alzheimer's disease. *Neuropsychiatric Diseases and Treatment* 2016; 12:869–875; https://doi.org/10.2147/NDT.S104886 (public access version available at www.ncbi.nlm.nih.gov/pmc/articles/PMC4841431).
4   Fornazzari L, Castle T, Nadkarni S, *et al.* Preservation of episodic musical memory in a pianist with Alzheimer's disease. *Neurology* 2006; 66:610–611; https://doi.org/10.1212/01.WNL.0000198242.13411.FB.
5   Levitin D. *This Is Your Brain on Music: The Science of a Human Obsession*. Dutton, 2006.
6   Münte TF, Altenmüller E and Jüncke J. The musician's brain as a model of neuroplasticity. *Nature Reviews Neuroscience* 2002; 3:473–478; https://doi.org/10.1038/nrn843.
7   Moreira SV, dos Reis Justi FR and Moreira M. Can musical intervention improve memory in Alzheimer's disease? Evidence from a systematic review. *Dementia & Neuropsychologia* 2018; 12:133–142; https://doi.org/10.1590/1980-57642018dn12-020005 (public access version available at www.ncbi.nlm.nih.gov/pmc/articles/PMC6022981).

16 IT'S ONLY SCARY IF YOU LOOK DOWN

Very early in my career, long before the advent of donepezil (Aricept) and other medications for treating the cognitive symptoms of Alzheimer's, a middle-aged woman came to see me for a second opinion. She had mild but troubling symptoms of cognitive impairment and had seen another neurologist who made a diagnosis of Alzheimer's disease. She had already had all the appropriate testing to exclude treatable mimics of dementia, and those tests were normal. Cognitive testing had shown some very subtle impairment of verbal memory and visual–spatial processing. I told her that she might indeed have very early Alzheimer's disease, but it was impossible for me to make that diagnosis with certainty. There were no tests to make a firm diagnosis of Alzheimer's at that time, other than a post-mortem examination of brain tissue. A few months later, I learned that she had taken her own life.

The memory of that patient has haunted me ever since. Now we have methods to make a firm diagnosis of Alzheimer's disease, even before cognitive symptoms start. We also know that the early stages of Alzheimer's disease can last many years, and that there are interventions that can slow progression of the disease if started early. My hope, both as a neurologist and as a person with Alzheimer's disease, is that, if we neurologists can learn to slow the progression of the disease even more, increase the years of relatively mild cognitive impairment, and postpone the awful end-stage, we patients may have a chance to die of other natural causes first. It would be wonderful if we could reach the point that considering suicide would not be necessary.

Climbing the steep trail up the face of Beacon Rock, it's easy enough to look straight ahead into the scenic surroundings and avoid the rail-side view looking down the sheer drop to the river below. I don't have a particular fear of heights, but I can appreciate that sometimes in life our view can take a precipitous drop down a scary slope. Sometimes a disturbing dream, a mood, a moment of forgetfulness or a depressive dip draws me in, takes my mind's eye to the trail's edge of this Alzheimer's path and I can't help but look down. It's an unsettling glimpse into the abyss.

Because early-stage Alzheimer's like mine ranges from no symptoms to relatively mild ones, I generally don't dwell on the darker aspects of late-stage Alzheimer's. But I know them well – I shared that difficult descent with my patients and their families for years as they coped with the changes and losses that Alzheimer's imposed as it advanced. The erosion of cognitive function and eventual loss of all memory, distant and recent. The inability to recognize loved ones; the potential for anger and lashing out; the loss of control, both physical and emotional. The depression, apathy and resignation. There is no dearth of books, no shortage of movie and media images that lay bare the indignities and losses of advanced Alzheimer's.

I am a neurologist, not a psychiatrist or psychologist. But, in my experience, someone's fear of the future as they come to terms with a diagnosis can often be debilitating beyond the burden of the physical illness itself. This is especially true for Alzheimer's disease because it is a neurodegenerative disease – it attacks the brain, and that alone is terrifying for most people. Compounding the fear is that, since the day the disease was formally identified more than 100 years ago, the only face of Alzheimer's has been that of the pitied, addled old person with advanced dementia. Everyone knows what that looks like, if not firsthand then from books, movies and other people's stories, and nobody wants to end up that way. Fear of that projected future hijacks any thinking about the present and its realistic possibilities.

An older man in his eighties, the proud patriarch of his family and a highly successful businessman, once came to see me about some mild memory issues. He passed the neurological exams and we both agreed that his memory issues could well be purely related to his advanced age. However, early-stage, pre-symptomatic Alzheimer's couldn't be ruled out. By this time, some potentially useful drugs were now available, and I explained that one particular medication often used to treat Alzheimer's might have a beneficial effect and might be worth trying to improve his memory function. He was incensed at the suggestion. He was adamant that he didn't have Alzheimer's, and he didn't want to take anything that was even faintly associated with Alzheimer's because it might suggest that he did. He stormed out of my office. Anger is sometimes a different face of fear.

Fear has kept countless others from exploring available options at the earliest sign of impairment, or kept them from sharing their diagnosis with family, which leaves them alone to manage their growing fear and the Alzheimer's symptoms as their cognitive impairment progresses. And, most devastating, fear has driven individuals to end their lives prematurely, like the woman whose story I shared above, while they felt they could still control their choices about life and death. Even without a diagnosis, the fear of a strong genetic risk alone can trigger the panic about end-stage Alzheimer's. When we're talking about genetic risk factors for scary diseases, it's easy to shift from learning mode to freak-out mode in a split second – the moment the information gets scary and personal, it triggers a version of the brain's flight-or-fight response. One moment, we're tracking the bear, the next moment we're face to face with it and our instinct is to run. In general, the brain has a hard time dealing with ambiguity and uncertainty; its impulse is always to jump to conclusions that feel familiar, even when they aren't right. The startled brain does this all the more so, and in that instant skips logical reasoning in favor of reactivity. So the nuances of risk can be hard to process calmly, even those in which the genetic dice may actually roll completely in your favor.

Case in point: It bears repeating that having the APOE-4 allele does not mean that someone will get Alzheimer's. They are at increased risk, especially if they have two copies, but *many APOE-4 carriers never get the disease*. Other risk factors involving other gene mutations or health history are relevant, and that's why it's important to approach these kinds of findings carefully, and with professional guidance. Nonetheless, on social media and in online chatrooms, the cautionary note from the DNA testing lab encouraging people to consult a genetic counselor is easily lost in the wind of worry, and sometimes despair, expressed in posts by people who have just received troubling DNA news. In this public forum, far from the private, HIPPA[1]-protected domain of the doctor/patient conversation, the posts range widely, but the discussion is often fraught. Shortly after I learned about my genetic loading for Alzheimer's from the ancestry-search DNA analysis, I went online to a chatroom of others who had received similar news, to see what I might discover there – perhaps resources or helpful insights. Most people expressed feelings of surprise and concern. One person was so upset by the news that she had a single copy of APOE-4 that she was considering suicide. I am not generally active on social media, not one to post in conversation threads, but I had to

---

[1]   Health Insurance Portability and Accountability Act (HIPPA) – a US law
       that protects the confidentiality of medical records.

reply. I explained that, although her one copy of APOE-4 meant that she was at greater risk of getting Alzheimer's than if she had no copies, it was still more likely than not that she would never get it.

Not just on social media, but in society more generally, the fear-driven conversation about Alzheimer's – which is really about advanced Alzheimer's – makes the need for attention to early-stage Alzheimer's all the more urgent. Early diagnosis of Alzheimer's disease will allow for mitigating actions, whether they be lifestyle changes, new medications or both. Individually, as families, and in the larger sense, we all need to be unafraid to examine our fears, hold them up to the light, because doing so can open possibilities we otherwise don't know exist.

Fear is a normal human reaction to something that feels threatening, and it comes up in different ways at different times. Understanding it doesn't mean I'm immune to it. For me, the dark side of Alzheimer's emerges in my dreams. I don't dream every night, and I rarely recall them in detail, but when I do remember a dream, it is almost always disturbing. The settings vary but there are several recurrent themes, all having to do with the sense of loss of control. I can't find my way, can't problem-solve effectively and can't find help. Or I can't communicate clearly, and people are puzzled or concerned by my incompetence.

There are different variations, all related to this sense of loss of control. In the travel dream, I am on a trip, usually by myself. It can be in Africa, Paris, London or the east coast of the US. Usually I am lost, or I can't get to the train station or airport in time to catch my train or plane. There is no one to help me. I feel alone and helpless.

My school dreams come in several variations. I am back in school, not for the first time, but for some inexplicable reason I have decided to repeat high school or college or medical school or residency as the person I am now, a 69-year-old with early-stage Alzheimer's. Because of my cognitive impairment, I am unable to complete an assignment or I fail a course and can't graduate. In one variation, I get lost on campus and can't find my dorm. In another I forget to check my mailbox until the end of the year, and then I can't find the key. When I'm back in my residency, I don't know how to operate the electronic medical record. I realize I can't write a prescription because I have given up my medical license. The other residents and interns think I am the attending physician because I am forty years their senior, and they are puzzled and concerned by my incompetence.

I was halfway through my annual two-week teaching engagement in Tanzania, in January 2016, just before the Phase 3 trial began, when I realized I was dreaming more, probably because of my anti-malarial medication or the heat. And the dreams often were explicitly about issues with Alzheimer's. One night, I dreamt that I got lost in a parking structure after parking, and when I finally found my way out, I had the parking sticker with me that I should have left on the car. Apparently, this had potentially serious ramifications; police confronted me. I explained to them that I had forgotten to leave the pass on the car because I had Alzheimer's disease. Strange – but not surprising, given that I was becoming increasingly aware of my cognitive impairment.

My teaching seminars with the medical students and KCMC staff had gone smoothly, as always. It had been encouraging that I still had no trouble giving PowerPoint presentations or teaching at the bedside. But I noticed that I could understand almost nothing now at those morning reports. It seemed like I was listening to a foreign language. I concluded it was the same issue I had at home now during some large family dinners, when I'd have difficulty filling in missing words from context, even when the context was home and family, the most familiar one there could be.

The connection between my waking reality and the canvas of my unconscious in dreams isn't hard to fathom. It's a single canvas, after all, for any of us. The day bleeds through into the night, a microhemorrhage of anxiety from one medium to another, from neurons to nightmares.

At the same time, the reality of a day or moments in a day can be so encouraging. A sense of agency can be an antidote for fear. On the trip that Lois and I took to the Kilimanjaro region, our ambitious day hike was exciting for all the obvious reasons, but for me, in particular, it was especially encouraging. In our travels and in my exercise regimen at home, to know that my physical capacities are strong despite the mild cognitive impairments, gives me a way to channel my attention to what I *can* do. However that changes on any given day, for either of us, staying present to the moment has become one of the most valuable tools we both would discover. And dreams can change: recently I had my first pleasant dream in some time. I was walking through a familiar neighborhood of Paris heading to an appointment with a potential translator for this book. I awoke from this dream at peace and remarkably hopeful for the future.

I generally don't dwell on the dark aspects of late-stage Alzheimer's. Lois and I have a kind of pact: live in the present. It's a practice. We've taken the steps needed to prepare for practical matters we can anticipate. Otherwise, we ground ourselves in the now. For me, that means that I do everything I can to protect and cultivate my cognitive health and postpone the late stage of Alzheimer's disease. In addition to those big-brush lifestyle choices about exercise, diet and the rest, I've discovered that the small-brush details often deliver surprising rewards.

I was just a kid, maybe eight or nine years old, when my father gave me my first camera, a hand-cranked, black box that looked more like a handheld Model-T than the technological ancestor of the digital camera we pop in our pockets today. Our backyard became my backlot studio, where I'd shoot still-life battle scenes with my toy soldiers in the grass. As my interest grew, my dad built a darkroom over the garage, and by high school I was spending a lot of time in there developing my own film, making prints, getting hooked on the hobby. Forty-plus years later, just as my career trained me to see as a scientist and physician, my camera has trained my eye for a different kind of detail: life with a slower shutter speed and a focus on nature.

As it happens, creative activities and time in nature are both considered of therapeutic value in the context of things you can do that promote brain health. This has special significance in the scientific literature relative to the aging brain, to dementia and, specifically, to Alzheimer's, because the disease often damages the part of the brain that normally enables you to retrieve internal imagery and copy it. However, as one study noted, "people with Alzheimer's disease can continue to produce art by using their remaining strengths, such as color or composition instead of shapes or realism" and "Remarkably, art emerges in some patients even in the face of degenerative disease" [1].

I've found that the act of taking pictures has made me look more carefully at landscapes and wildlife, and that, especially in recent years, it helps my memory. I'll photograph a bird or animal that I can't identify, then set out to learn more about them through other sources. Sometimes the shot I get holds other surprises. A few years ago, a juvenile bald eagle (native to our area) happened to land on the wall in my backyard when, by chance, I had my camera with a long lens in hand. I was pleased enough to have captured the shot of this beautiful young raptor at such close range, but there was something more in store. In the photo, the eagle's right pupil, the one in the sun, is smaller than his left pupil. In humans and most mammals, if you shine a light in one eye, both pupils will constrict to the same degree. This is called the consensual pupillary response, and it's something that a neurologist checks for because the lack of it can indicate where a lesion may be in the brain. I wondered what it meant in a bird, and had to look it up, but it turns out that, in birds, the consensual pupillary response is only partial, or absent altogether.

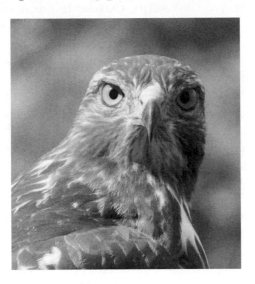

Juvenile bald eagle.

That might not seem like something to get excited about, this small discovery of something I didn't know before. But, just as a small upset has the power to distract from a good day, sometimes a small thing can set me right again, shift my attention to the wider, more satisfying view that lets me carry on.

Mentors are all around. Befitting his spaniel senses, Jack lives his life in mentor mode, a serial enthusiast, ready to be enthralled at any moment by a small thing. Or at least pleased. He can be in a deep snooze in the family room, and at the faintest sound of meal prep starting in the kitchen, he races to my side or to Lois' (especially if she's preparing chicken), determined to miss nothing. Every flick of my knife through a green pepper, carrot or broccoli floret is, for Jack, ripe with anticipation. He sits at full attention, in case a vegetable should accidentally-on-purpose tumble his way. He is also attentive to cheese-grating, cooked-chicken-slicing and watermelon-cutting, to name a few of his interests. We make sure that he is rarely disappointed. During meals, he stations himself under the table, seeming to know the difference between attentive and intrusive, but always alert, in stealth mode, ready for the moment that someone leaves the table for some reason and leaves their plate unattended; he jumps at the opportunity to assist in the clean-up. Lois notes that Jack actually gets very little people-food, certainly not enough to justify the amount of energy he puts into trying to get it. But he's a dog, she says, and he doesn't have a whole lot else to do, so perhaps he finds it worthwhile.

So I've learned to watch for the moments. Every tidbit feels worthwhile. Maybe it's a book I'm reading and enjoying, which I won't remember in any detail two weeks from now. Maybe it's Jack as he sniffs every shrub on our forest walk. Or the sight of Lois, earbuds in place as she listens to an audio book and fits the next piece into the jigsaw puzzle. Our kids and our grandkids. The lists and other planning for the next summer's San Juan sailing expedition with Henry and John. The conversation with a colleague about a new finding emerging in a clinical trial or neuroscience laboratory. The reality of a day, or a moment in a day, can be so encouraging.

One thing that is striking as you get near the top of Beacon Rock is to look down at the boat dock below. The boats tied up to it are so tiny you can hardly make them out. Looking down isn't always scary. It can also heighten your sense of gain in altitude. You can feel how far you've come. Even if it takes a conscious effort to do so, you can take the moment to savor that.

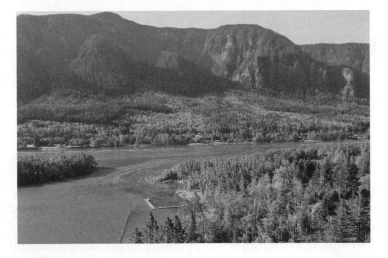

Looking down on the dock at the foot of Beacon Rock from near the summit.

Chapter-references

1 Cummings JL, Miller BL, Christensen DD, Cherry D. Creativity and dementia: emerging diagnostic and treatment methods for Alzheimer's disease. *CNS Spectrums* 2008; 13(2 Suppl. 2):1–22.

17 BEYOND DNA: FAMILY HISTORY RECONSIDERED

What makes us what we are? The old nature versus nurture debate isn't one anymore. We know that our genetic inheritance is only a part of what shapes us. We are, of course, shaped by our experiences throughout our lives, but perhaps most so when we are children. What we learn from our parents depends not only on their genes, but perhaps most strongly on cultural inheritance, the ideas, philosophies, literary preferences, religious beliefs, likes, dislikes and prejudices passed down from our ancestors and blended together into an ethical, artistic and intellectual amalgam.

So often in the Alzheimer's conversation, or that of any disease with genetic links, as the search for clarity around a diagnosis is paramount, discussion of family history brings parents and extended family into sharp view for that purpose alone – their DNA trail. Short of conclusive findings, then, memorable behaviors come under new scrutiny for evidence – in this case, for dementia. Could an elder's notorious forgetfulness or odd behavior have been a symptom of cognitive decline associated with Alzheimer's? What other patterns of behavior or health issues might suggest a genetic predisposition?

I heard this for years as a neurologist – I facilitated it in fact, this narrowing narrative aimed at unearthing a genetic inheritance. I didn't really think beyond the need to learn everything possible for a diagnosis, to provide a basis to plan treatment. When I first learned of my own genetic inheritance – that I carried two sets of the APOE-4 gene – that's exactly where my thoughts went, too. I soon realized that both of my parents had died of other health problems before they reached the age at which Alzheimer's symptoms might have emerged. I would never know whether, had they lived long enough, they would have developed dementia with the genetic hallmarks of Alzheimer's. I saw new significance in old family stories of elders whose erratic or odd behavior had raised a few eyebrows back in the day. This was clinically relevant; these family members became clinically relevant. There is nothing wrong with that. But they deserve better.

These days, as I think more deliberately about the past to exercise my memory, I find myself reflecting on it in new ways. I've come to appreciate the concept of genetic inheritance in a fuller way. Just as surely as my brown eyes, my wiry build and my APOE-4 genes represent genetic influences, so do many of the qualities and traits that have defined my life.

My father, Zack Gibbs, was a scientist not by training, but by nature. He embodied the scientist's intense curiosity, critical thinking and love of hands-on experimentation, and he became an incredible mentor in my scientific education. An engineer, he encouraged me to build my own toys and not expect store-bought ones. When I ran into design issues, he would usually let me fail on my own, and then help me figure out how to improve the design. There was the wooden go-cart I built when I was about eight years old. I assembled the chassis with nails, only to have the whole thing fall apart after a few bumpy runs down a hill. My father showed me where the stresses were occurring and how to reinforce those points with appropriately sized bolts, nuts and washers. As I got a little older, he led me through more sophisticated experiments, mostly centered around electricity – and pretty dangerous, all things considered. But I learned at a very early age that risk must be managed and that lab technique must be meticulous.

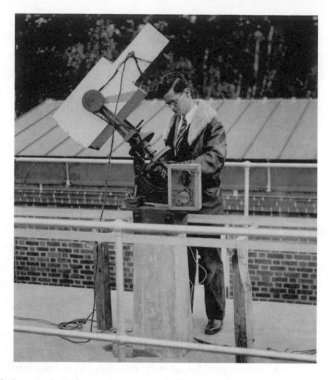

My father Zack Gibbs at the Harvard Observatory. At age 28, he was already an avid amateur photographer. I believe he took this photo himself.

All through my middle-school years, my father and I went to weekly public lectures given by professors at nearby Cal Tech. By the end of middle school, there was no doubt that I wanted to be a scientist. I think the single most important attribute I got from my father was the enjoyment of being curious – discovering new things, broadening my horizons, learning to love science. My childhood experience, guided by my father, gave me the tools I would use in the years ahead to build a career and life as a scientist, a physician, and a father myself.

Although my mother only briefly attended college, she was an avid reader and loved music. She was an excellent amateur pianist, and she encouraged me early in life to make music. I took to it with gusto, starting to compose music in fourth grade, even before I had started piano lessons. I remember playing a piece at school that I had written and annotated on musical staff paper with my mother's help. The following year, I started piano lessons that continued on and off through college. I added a few additional instruments – guitar, saxophone, harmonica and trumpet over the years – eventually even playing lead electric guitar in a high school rock band. Music continues to be a big part of my life. While there was nothing gentle about our rock band repertoire, I think of my mother's gift of music as just part of the way she helped me shape my softer sides. She was a complicated person, reserved and not the soft-fuzzy emotionally expressive type of personality, but her appreciation for beauty, be it in music, the fine arts or her beloved garden, found its receptors in me.

And so on. My sisters and my late Uncle Fred. Lois and our kids and grandkids. As much as any genes I was dealt at conception, they have made me who I am. When I consider the prescriptive lifestyle choices that protect the brain and fight against the Alzheimer's disease processes, and what happens when you set out to take them from page to practice, none of that happens in a vacuum. Lois and our kids, especially, shape my every experience.

Lois and I have been partners now for fifty-one years and married for forty-eight of them. Her career path as a librarian was no accident – she has always been very organized and methodical, and she has tried for our entire life together to get some of that need for organization to rub off on me, with only limited success. But perseverance is an enduring trait of hers, and her patience in keeping after me to learn planning and time-management skills threads through any success I might claim as my own, especially

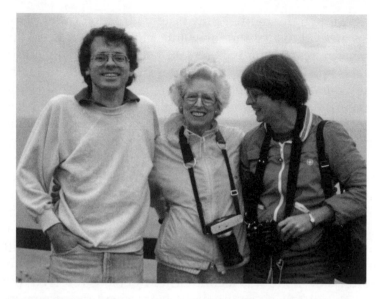

My mother, sister Nancy and me in 1982. My sister Mollie took
the photo.

now that I'm losing my ability to make plans and multitask
as I slip farther into the fog of Alzheimer's. I have loved to
read all my life, but Lois is the reason I have successfully kept reading throughout this experience. Her voracious
reading habit – upwards of 300 books a year – her enthusiasm for sharing recommendations and her librarian's ease
as a guide to other resources meant she got me hooked on
the reading challenges of Goodreads. When I completely
lost my ability to read during my ARIA episode, she urged
me to try audiobooks, and that worked. I was surprised
that, even though I couldn't visually decipher written text,
I had no trouble understanding a book that was read to
me. If not for Lois' keen eye on the subtext of life after our
dog died, leaving us melancholy empty-nesters and dogless
"dog-people," my own characteristic hesitation might easily have allowed the losses to color our life longer. Instead:
Jack!

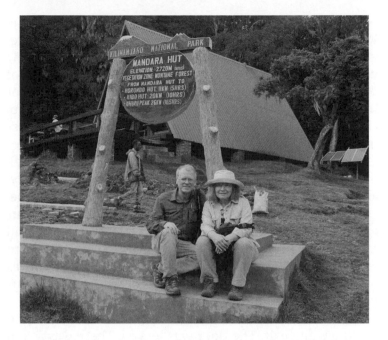

Lois and me on our day hike to the Mandara Hut on Mt. Kilimanjaro. Photo in author's collection.

Our kids stay in touch, and I am able to read and talk and play with my grandchildren (if not always in person then via video chats) – how much leaner my prescriptive strategies for intellectual stimulation and social interaction would be without them to bolster my defenses.

The old friends who've stayed friends draw long threads through our shared history, each one a world of experience that has shaped what I know and how I understand things, from science to sailing.

I recently visited my friend R. in a skilled nursing facility. R. is six or seven years older than me. He was one of the partners in the neurology group practice that I joined after I completed my neurology residency in 1989. He was always available to answer my questions about a perplexing patient or just the nuts and bolts of the neurology practice. We grew to be good friends and nearly always lunched together for the next twenty-one years. Over the last few years, his health has worsened due to a combination of chronic physical ailments. Throughout all this, he has kept his wry sense of humor and remained cognitively sharp. He still does some consulting work as an expert witness in medico-legal cases. We have continued to get together for lunch every few months. About a month ago, he developed a severe infection, an abscess that required surgery, a three-week hospital stay and an extended recovery period in the skilled nursing facility. We spent a great hour exchanging notes on our respective families, dogs and neurological problems, and we agreed that being able to examine our own issues dispassionately through the eyes of neurologists was a useful coping technique, allowing us both to assess our futures with some equanimity.

As I left his room, I found my way to the door leading to the stairs and exit. The door was locked. There was a sign that read "Do not assist patients trying to leave the facility." I looked around to check that no potential escapees were lurking nearby. All clear. I then read the instructions for unlocking the door. I was to punch in a series of six numbers and one symbol in reverse order. Okay, I thought, I can do this. I tried four times and failed. I finally asked a passing nurse to help me. When I got home, I texted R., telling him that I had flunked the cognitive eligibility test for leaving his facility. He texted back: *LOL*. And I did. I don't know how that might have registered on a real-time functional MRI brain scan, but I do know that, at what could easily have been a frustrating, embarrassing experience that dogged me for days, we laughed and the moment stuck, without the sting.

At the end of the day, as Rudy Tanzi noted, we can alter our gene expression programs "through daily conscious choices and experiences." Beyond family, I recognize the "inheritance" of close friends and colleagues whose qualities and traits shape my response to Alzheimer's and other life challenges – opportunities, too. They have all been active partners in my daily choices and experiences all my life. And in conversations with those who are on their own path with this disease, whether they have Alzheimer's themselves or have a family member or friend with it, it is heartening to refocus beyond genetic markers and, instead, on the wholeness of these individuals, and ourselves as well. I feel my mood shift when I appreciate the colorations of character and values they passed on to me, a transference that goes on all around us, all the time, by way of these essential others in our lives. From them and from one another, we may draw insight, endurance, courage, compassion or just the ability to laugh in the moment. And perhaps create a legacy of our own.

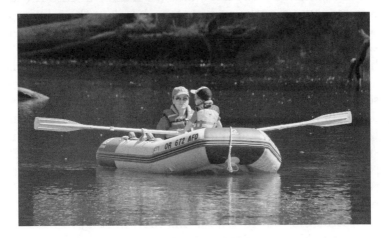

My son teaching his son how to row.

18 NEWS AT 5: RETIRED NEUROLOGIST BATTLES ALZHEIMER'S

Lois pushed 'pause' on her audiobook and slipped off her earbuds so she could answer the phone. Flavia de Luce could wait. The name on caller ID announced it was a longtime acquaintance we see occasionally when we cross paths on day hikes in the backwoods Oregon region where she lives. It was mid-March and we hadn't been out that way for some months, waiting for a break in the rainy season. She and Lois exchanged a few cheerful words. Then she asked after the family and Jack – it turned out she'd happened to be watching the local TV news and the image of an English Cocker Spaniel like Jack flashed on the screen and caught her attention. (He is a very handsome dog.) Then she had noticed my face on the screen and realized it *was* Jack. Then she saw the screen caption on the story – RETIRED NEUROLOGIST BATTLES ALZHEIMER'S [1]. And in that second, she was astonished to realize that the retired neurologist battling Alzheimer's was me. She'd picked up the phone and called.

In the days that followed, this private story of ours became a public one. People in the neighborhood, others I knew but didn't see often, and others who'd seen me on the nightly news would call or stop by – often with condolences on the grim future they imagined in store for me and for us, which could be awkward since I wasn't there yet. In fact, most stories about people with Alzheimer's are about those with moderate to severe stages of the disease. There is very little out there, very little in publicized research and very little in the public eye at all, about early-stage Alzheimer's, the mostly asymptomatic years before the onset of the neurodegeneration and cognitive decline that becomes noticeable. There is even less about anyone in early-stage Alzheimer's like myself, and measures they are taking that may slow the progression of the disease and buy themselves some precious time.

We all know that Alzheimer's robs us of the future we hoped for. But, in the absence of attention to the risk factors, and this earliest stage of the disease and the potential for positive interventions, our silence allows Alzheimer's to rob us of even more – possibly years more.

I am optimistic that we will be able to prevent and even cure Alzheimer's disease – probably not in my lifetime, but almost certainly for my children's generation. It will take a huge effort. It will take billions more dollars for research. And it will take tens or even hundreds of thousands of volunteers to participate in research studies, people who currently have Alzheimer's, and others who don't yet have symptoms of cognitive impairment but who have a family history of Alzheimer's, carry an APOE-4 gene or have other risk factors for the disease. It will take expanding research to include populations that have been long underrepresented in studies – African American and Latino, specifically [2]. All of these volunteers will be the real heroes who lead to the cure.

We need those who can to press for public policy that not only supports research for treatment and cure, but ensures that all may access these advances. Although it is currently illegal to deny healthcare coverage for people who have tested positive for brain amyloid, it may be difficult or impossible to obtain long-term care insurance once that information is available. Some people worry about potential family issues and social stigma that might be associated with a positive diagnosis. All of these are significant concerns, difficult to sort out quickly or easily. But they only add urgency to the need for public policy that protects us and advances research for effective treatment. Silence works against progress, and against us.

We each do what we can. That's going to look different depending on who you are and how Alzheimer's lands in your life. One thing we can do is to take the private battle public.

The last time I was in touch with Greg O'Brien, his body and his faculties were failing in so many ways, but his spirit remained outsized. He was as articulate as ever – he is a journalist, after all – and he sent me a link to a recent article he wrote for *Psychology Today* about the surviving caregivers of a few of his friends who have died recently from Alzheimer's [3]. It's not a maudlin essay. It's actually hopeful, and it's a testament to his Irish resolve and the resolve of the spouses of his friends. He is a wonderful and articulate advocate for Alzheimer's awareness and action, and he's still going strong.

I'm no journalist, and it took some time for me to feel I could speak, or write, beyond medical conferences and journals. I was able to step out of my comfort zone when it occurred to me that the longer I waited to do so, the less likely I'd be able to put thoughts to page. However personal my medical battle against Alzheimer's, more than anything now I've committed to the larger one. I am battling its power to avert our gaze, to muzzle the potential of science and medicine to make more dramatic strides, to intimidate and silence us and, in doing so, have us fail to address the challenges and promise that early diagnosis and treatment may hold.

When I decided to go public with my story for the first time, in that television interview, I was basically deciding to take the "fight" public – not to gain attention for myself, but to heighten awareness of the situation that is developing right now for millions of others, and to do everything possible to stir conversation and action around it. Silence works against progress; it works against us.

Chapter-references

1   LaBrecque J. Retired neurologist with Alzheimer's shares importance of early awareness. *KATU News* March 26, 2019; https://katu.com/news/local/retired-neurologist-with-alzheimers-shares-importance-of-early-awareness.

2   Staples GB. Opinion: why having more Blacks, Latinos in Alzheimer's trials is vital. *The Atlanta Journal-Constitution* July 23, 2020; www.ajc.com/life/opinion-why-having-more-blacks-latinos-in-alzheimers-trials-is-vital/AAP65TZYIJGZDIVW467HLW6654.

3   O'Brien G. Confessions of a caregiver. *Psychology Today* January 16, 2020; www.psychologytoday.com/us/blog/pluto/202001/confessions-caregiver.

19 THE FOREST, THE TREES AND THE GROUND BENEATH MY FEET

Lois could hear the familiar Bach prelude wafting upstairs from the piano and she was pleased that I was playing, since I usually wait until she's out with Jack to do so. Jack has a tendency to howl or try to climb in my lap, though whether that is a complaint or a desire to perform a duet, we don't know. Our daughter Susannah was in for a visit, and Jack wasn't howling, probably distracted. But, as Lois listened, she noticed the prelude sounded a bit halting, with a few mistakes. She paused, worried in that moment, for the first time, that Alzheimer's might be showing itself this way, and came downstairs to look in on me. She was relieved to discover it wasn't me at all – it was Susannah, the flutist in the family. Susannah rarely plays piano at all anymore, except to join Elizabeth for their hilarious, haphazard rendition of Christmas carols for our family gathering. But there she was, picking her way through the sheet music, playing for fun.

Lois keeps a good game face, but I know she watches for subtle changes, as do I. My continued independence is important to both of us. Lois knows it goes to the heart of my being and our life together. I've traveled the world for my work and volunteer commitments; we've traveled together to share adventures; and every August when I join Henry and John for our San Juan sailing expedition, I've always been in charge of the planning. It's tradition, a high point of the summer, not just for us sailors but for Lois, too – a generous expanse of that hard-earned solitary splendor.

Her independence is just as important to us both. In the ARIA episode, when I suddenly lost my ability to read and spiraled down until doctors were able to turn the situation around, it was Lois who instantly confronted the implications of this new impairment. Among other things, the safety issues it raised were paramount. Safety concerns would change everything about my independence going forward – and hers, too. If I were unable to read and get around safely on my own, my annual trips to Tanzania and other international commitments would be out of the question. Even the simplest trips to the grocery store or other routine errands would be hazardous if I were unable to read street names or signs or labels. The impact on daily life of suddenly and permanently not being able to read or write would be wide ranging, affecting forms of communication with friends and family, in addition to the impact on Alzheimer's-related work. Talks and presentations would no longer be possible without being able to rely on notes. Reading the mail, paying bills and keeping up with emails would no longer be possible. Working crossword puzzles, reading for pleasure, researching and ordering things, among many other facets of daily life, would no longer be possible. I would have been completely dependent on someone else to either do these things or provide assistance. Lois had to fast-forward by herself to that imagined watershed moment; for those few weeks that my brain could no longer read, I was caught in the confusion itself, not in the awareness of what it meant. Once recovered – thankfully recovered – months later, I resumed my vigilance, reminded that any small slip might turn out to be the one that signaled the new normal that Alzheimer's would impose.

The concern was reasonable. Before the ARIA episode, but well into the period of time since I'd been diagnosed with early-stage Alzheimer's, my scores on the Montreal Cognitive Assessment (MOCA) hovered around 27 to 29. I don't think I ever scored a perfect 30. During my adverse reaction in the drug trial and the several months of confusion that followed, my MOCA score dropped to 20, in the dementia range. But within six months after I had fully recovered, my score was back up to 27. Since then, there has been a gradual drop off in my MOCA score. It was 25 when I was last tested six months ago. This was entirely due to not being able to recall any of the five words after five minutes. This correlates nicely with the more extensive cognitive testing that I have had, which shows my cognitive impairment as largely confined to verbal memory.

It's great that I am still testing as well as I am. On the MOCA, I am still in the mild cognitive impairment range, and I find that reassuring as I know that the Alzheimer's pathology is proceeding in my brain. I have seen the tau-containing neurofibrillary tangles spreading on the PET scan of my brain. Those horses are stomping their feet, anxious to get out of the barn. I'm counting on my cognitive reserve and aggressive lifestyle modifications to keep those horses confined for as long as possible.

I don't mention every little thing to Lois and she doesn't constantly quiz me. But she is no less aware, I am sure. Very little escapes her notice around this house and in the family, and what she doesn't see, she seems to intuit. Sometime after last summer's week-long San Juan sailing trip, Henry had mentioned in passing to Lois one day that he could tell no difference in my ability to navigate. It was reassuring to her that things were still going well with the sailing trips.

Every year I look forward to planning several annual trips, the first to Tanzania in the spring to visit my colleagues at the hospital and my old friend William Howlett, who continues his work as the head of neurology at the hospital there. Then Lois and I plan some kind of

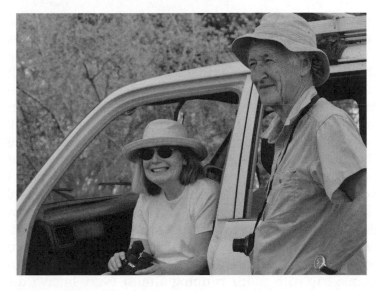

Lois and my friend Dr. William Howlett on a photo safari in Tanzania.
Dr. Howlett has worked as a neurologist in Africa since the 1980s.
He was one of the first to describe the neurological complications of
HIV/AIDS.

travel adventure for late spring or early summer; this year
it would be to explore Shetland, Orkney, and the Faroe
Islands and Iceland, Covid permitting. An international
conference – sometimes two – in the summer, and then
in August the sailing trip with John and Henry. I especially looked forward to the upcoming trip to Tanzania,
assuming it might be my last opportunity to spend time
on the ground there with friends, in the company of
Mt. Kilimanjaro. We email regularly, but there is nothing
like being there.

Although I have made that trip to Tanzania by myself
almost yearly for the last twelve years, I recognize that my
ability to problem-solve for travel irregularities is probably not as robust as it once was. Over the past six months,
I've noticed increasing problems with my short-term

memory. I just couldn't remember whether something had happened earlier in the day, yesterday, or even last week. I couldn't seem to place events onto the time scale of my recent history, and time seemed to be passing much more rapidly. I think that, because I don't remember the details of what I have done earlier in the day or earlier in the week, my sense of the passage of time has been altered.

I kept that in mind while arranging this trip. I made plans to be met at the airport in Tanzania by a driver, and I wouldn't venture out on my own. On the way home, I would stop in London for a few days. I had originally planned to take the train on a day trip to Portsmouth to visit the Portsmouth Historic Dockyard and see the eighteenth-century battleships of the British Royal Navy. I have never been to Portsmouth, and although it seems to be a simple trip with trains running almost every hour, I decided to forgo the Portsmouth side trip and restrict my stay to the South Kensington neighborhood right around the Victoria and Albert Museum and the Natural History Museum. Less chance for getting lost or disoriented. Strategies and tactics.

Over the years, the planning alone has become a ritual – challenging and, in recent years, reassuring that I could still do it. Any thoughts otherwise feel premature for the time being.

There has been a very gradual worsening in cognitive impairment that is hardly perceptible. Talking this over with Lois, we agree that the most noticeable change has been less fluid speech. I will start a sentence and then divert to a related thought, sometimes without completing the thought I started with. There also seems to be a slight worsening in my ability to understand what is being said to me. It appears to be a processing-speed problem. When Lois starts to say something to me, I may not understand what she is saying, and I often ask her to say it again. However, if I pause for a moment or two, often I can process and understand what she has just said. Once she has my attention, I usually have no further trouble with that conversation. It's just at the start. And my balance is getting just a little worse, mostly still just on the stairs. This is most likely due to further worsening of proprioception.

Strategies and tactics on the home front include simple things like a pill organizer. Each Saturday night, I fill the pill organizer for the next week. There are fourteen compartments, one a.m. and one p.m. for each day. I must concentrate on the task at hand and not think of anything else while I do this, as on more than one occasion I have forgotten one of the pills. As a double-check at the end, I count them. Good mental exercise anyway. Mnemonics help me with the increasing problem recalling names. It's something like tinkering with electrical connections in the experiments I used to do as a kid with my father. Only now I'm hotwiring my brain for names. So, to recall my neighbor Walt's name, I start with the thought of Disneyland, which gets me to Walt Disney, which lights up the synapses to Walt my neighbor. My brain recalls my colleague, Dr. Lisa Silbert, by name only after starting with the thought of a hazelnut (the state nut of Oregon), then filbert (the other name for hazelnuts) – then Silbert. Many people use mnemonics to enhance their memory skills, and it's interesting to think how a seemingly convoluted neural processing sequence could be considered an advantage – until you imagine how that circuitry enables a brain like mine to skirt the plaques and tangles to make the needed connection. At the same time, I'm glad I can relegate some organizational tasks to sticky notes and digital assistants and save my bandwidth for other things.

I think, in the early stages of Alzheimer's disease, most people are aware of their cognitive issues, but some may be in denial and unwilling to admit to them. I saw this in some of my patients. That makes it more difficult to detect a disease process that could be addressed sooner rather than later. As a neurologist, I used to feel that people in the moderate and late stages were sometimes oblivious to their cognitive problems, but I suspect that may not be true. Certainly, agitation and behavioral problems are common in the late stages, and I wonder whether those issues may be in part caused by fear and frustration with cognitive limitations. Ask me again in a few years.

While I do keep track of my cognitive changes, I am not obsessively waiting for some new symptom. When I do notice something new, it may get my attention, and it can be a little scary. I can still balance the checkbook, sometimes on the first try. But a month or two ago, I had a bad day when it took five tries before getting it right, and the differences each time were huge. That was something new and alarming. But these issues to some extent wax and wane. Sometimes when I can't think of a name – that of a colleague, for instance – I'll run through a mental list of other colleagues and occasionally I will draw repeated blanks. Other times, I can remember names pretty well.

Technology presents its own set of challenges for any of us, especially those of us who aren't digital natives as our children and grandchildren are. Our laptops, smartphones, e-readers and tablets are helpful – if not essential – to those whose minds aren't as sharp as they once were, and incredibly frustrating, with frequent changes, updates and new learning required. Like most people we know who are our age, we depend on calendars, notes, reminders, a quick search for missing bits of information, on phones or tablets or laptops. However, changes to familiar computer programs can just be impenetrable, and organizing files and bookmarks is tricky at the best of times. Especially for me. Electronic appliances can be hard to learn to operate. We only barely know how to operate our smart TV; the remote is a bit mystifying at times. Lois points out that I have never mastered the timer on our kitchen range. Challenges relating to technology make up an area where we have taken advantage of our younger family members' expertise. Asking for help can be hard. On the other hand, any particular glitch is as likely to be a generational thing as an Alzheimer's thing, and our adult children and their spouses have graciously provided tech help and advice when needed. As a result, I've gotten over most of my self-consciousness about asking.

In the meantime, I don't dwell on these matters. I don't obsess about measuring my decline. I do occasionally take the smartphone test that I was using during the exercise study, but my feeling is that it is relatively insensitive, especially to impairment of verbal memory. Every six months, I complete an online questionnaire for the Brain Health Registry that includes some cognitive tests, but I don't know how my results compare to my previous answers. I don't usually communicate with my doctors except at yearly or, in some cases, twice-yearly appointments. Those evaluations confirm that I continue to do remarkably well from a cognitive standpoint, and I look at it optimistically that my cognitive decline has been as slow as it has. I would like to think that this is due at least in part to the lifestyle changes I have adopted. Although I can't be certain, the possibility helps motivate me to stay the course each day.

Because I have had so little cognitive deterioration, it is easy to forget that I am headed for disaster in the future. I think it is healthy to not dwell on the future, as long as one is prepared, which Lois and I are, in all practical ways – as well as we can be. Equanimity can be harder as a family, since each of us relates to the disease and its impact differently. We don't really talk in depth about my Alzheimer's, as a family. One of my daughters mentioned that she'd been surprised to learn one particular detail for the first time in something I wrote that appeared in the *New York Times*. I think our children may feel that we don't keep them up to date on symptoms and developments to keep them from worrying. Though we phone and see them frequently, sometimes every day, we don't necessarily relate all the ups and downs of daily life – the minor slip of memory, a gate accidentally left open, or a hose not completely turned off. We don't dwell on bad news, but we would certainly keep them informed of any significant worrisome developments. Our conversations are largely focused on their more active and interesting lives, careers, families and their households, which, like ours, are not entirely free of mishaps from time to time – some worth mentioning, and others not. They are busy people, early in their own careers, caring for young children or pets, and dealing with home maintenance issues. We do not want them to worry about us. That is natural for parents. The time may come when we will ask more of them, for moral support or companionship or care, through the process of Alzheimer's or aging, and we trust that they will be available, caring and resilient, as they have proven to be in times of distress all through our lives. We're a family of planners, so naturally we would all be more comfortable if we had a timetable and could plan ahead what would be required at each step, but we don't have that. There's a lot that we – us as a family and, in the broader sense, those in science and medicine – don't know, so it's hard to be prepared with specific plans. At this point, no one knows how long this earlier, higher- functioning stage will last, and what the circumstances will be when, and if, later-stage care is needed. What is known is that this early stage is potentially quite a long period of time and there aren't a lot of significant changes occurring regularly. It's not so much an intent to be secretive – there just isn't anything much to report.

Day to day, I fare better if I train my attention to stay present to the moment. I do have down days when I don't feel very good and feel more flustered than usual. We all have days like that. I've had enough of them in life, well before Alzheimer's, to know that one down day doesn't necessarily mean the next day will be the same. Even with Alzheimer's, I've experienced coming through hard days and eventually feeling better, I remind myself. I felt crummy the morning I went into the research center for the dosing study for the cognitive-enhancing botanical compound. But then I thought about the list of contributing factors, including that I'd been fasting for twelve hours, had had no caffeine for three days, and was off my walking routine. I also thought about the up-side: while there, I edited drafts for several hours and read forty or so pages of *Slaughterhouse-Five*. I've just realized there are going to be cycles, and, so far, there has not been an overall linear trend that's downward and frightening.

Neuropsychologists have extensive batteries of cognitive tests that can accurately home in on the part of the brain that may be damaged in a patient with cognitive impairment. These tests can take an hour or even more to administer, so they generally aren't practical for screening purposes. There are at least three screening tests that are commonly used by neurologists to get a rough idea whether a patient has cognitive impairment, and even these relatively short tests may give a hint to the part of the brain that is in distress. They are all based on a perfect score of 30, and anything lower than 26 is generally considered to be abnormal.

When I first started seeing dementia patients in 1989, none of these tests was widely available. Most of us had our own screening questions, such as: "Tell me the date today"; "What place is this?"; "What time is it?"; "Name the last five presidents." I would give them three words to remember and ask them again in five minutes. I would have them copy a complex figure. These questions were not standardized, and it was difficult to interpret the results.

The first of the commonly used screening tests was the Mini-Mental State Exam (MMSE). It was first published in 1975, but it was protected by copyright. Nevertheless, most of us were using it by the mid-1990s, largely because one of the big drug companies provided it as a give-away. It's a good screening test, but it has been criticized as being relatively insensitive. It is pretty easy to score above 26, and it seemed to miss early cases of dementia.

Late in my career, I switched over to using two newer tests, the St. Louis University Mental Status Test (SLUMS) and the MOCA. I think they are both more sensitive than the MMSE. I especially like the MOCA because it comes in three forms with different words to remember, different number sequences to recall, different animals to name, etc. This helps to minimize learning bias. After subjects have taken the same test repeatedly, they begin to learn the responses, especially if their cognitive problem is mild. I still score a perfect 30 almost every time I am given the MMSE because I gave it almost daily for fifteen years or so and I know all the answers. On the MOCA, I scored 29 when I first started getting regular testing in 2015, but at my last test six months ago, my score had dropped to 25. My neurologist rotates through the three forms of the test so I can't remember the answers from one time to the next.

The MOCA starts out with three tests of visual–spatial processing. In the trail-making test, you are asked to connect ten small circles in the right order starting at 1, then A, then 2, then B etc. Then you have to copy a complex figure. Then you're asked to draw a clock face with the numbers and show the hands pointing to a specific time. Next, you're asked to name drawings of three animals. Then memory is tested by asking you to learn five words. They are spoken to you, then five minutes later you're asked to recall them. Attention is tested by asking you to repeat a list of five digits forward and three digits backward, doing serial subtractions, and then tapping a finger on the table every time you hear a specific letter as a random group of letters is recited. Language is tested by having you repeat two fairly complex sentences. There is a brief test of the ability to understand abstract relationships between words. Finally, orientation is tested, much like with the MMSE.

Of course, I can't give myself these tests. The answers are included with the questions. There are online cognitive tests. I have tried a few of them, including a new one that I used as part of a clinical trial. I really haven't found any of these computerized tests to be very sensitive to my fairly isolated deficiency in verbal memory.

At the other end of the spectrum from these tests that aim for a granular view of cognitive impairment is a simpler, more descriptive approach shared by noted pioneer in geriatric psychiatry Dr. Gene Cohen, who worked extensively with patients who had Alzheimer's. Asked to explain how someone's lucidity, or clarity of mind, changes with different stages of Alzheimer's disease, he offered this analogy: "For healthy persons, their lucidity allows them to see the forest. For persons in the mild stage of AD [Alzheimer's disease], they can no longer see the forest, just some trees. For persons in the moderate stage of AD, they can no longer see the trees, just some branches. For persons in the severe stage of AD, they can no longer see the branches, just a blurr" [1].

By that measure, I'm relieved to say that at this point in my own Alzheimer's experience, most days I can still see the forest, and always the trees, but, perhaps even more important to me, I can focus on the ground beneath my feet and feel fully present to life.

As it turned out, in the course of writing this book, in the matter of a few weeks between paragraphs, the coronavirus pandemic struck. Among effects far worse than canceled travel plans in early spring of 2020, all international travel was off for everyone for the foreseeable future. Even when travel restrictions eventually ease, I can't be certain I'll be in a position a year from now to take on the demands of that kind of travel, so this may prove the abrupt end to those traditions. Professional conferences have all been shifted to virtual platforms, no gatherings. And I'm grateful that the curb on travel, or even local forays under quarantine measures, are the only hardship for us personally at this point, when people are suffering more awful consequences every day all around us. One day, a friend and I are talking about the pandemic, about the swift spread here and everywhere, and the suddenness with which the coronavirus strikes and kills. Death comes so unexpectedly. I've grown accustomed to speaking of the predictability of Alzheimer's, the eventual end-stage extreme, acknowledging that as my inevitable fate and expressing a preference that my family be spared that. "Alzheimer's will kill me if something else doesn't get me first, which I hope it does," I've said casually at times. My friend reminds me of those words and how they play in the current coronavirus context.

"Be careful what you wish for," she says.

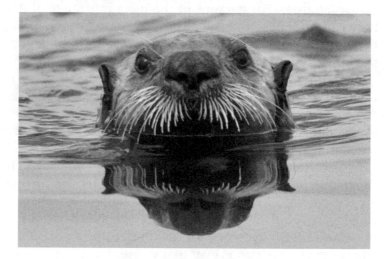

Sea otter off one of the Aleutian Islands.

I'm struck by the irony of it now: that the long-range Alzheimer's prognosis I refer to – a statistically predictable death after a period of sharp decline in my mental and physical function – assumes the luxury of time. The pandemic has made us all rethink that. Today, like everyone else I know, I'm taking all possible protective measures against the virus, acting with an abundance of caution, for my family's safety and that of others. And myself. I'm actually not ready to go. Timing is everything. And life is good.

Chapter-reference

1   Miller WL, Cohen GD. *Sky Above Clouds: Finding Our Way through Creativity, Aging and Illness*. Oxford University Press, 2016, p. 130.

20 WHAT'S IN A NAME? ALZHEIMER'S REIMAGINED

Early in my career, when I chose to step away from research and devote my career to clinical neurology, one of the most compelling reasons was how much I loved working directly with patients, able to bring cutting-edge medical approaches to them and see the difference these made in their lives. When I was in medical school, somebody once told me that his father had been a neurologist but had left to go into research because patients were disheartening – there was so little to be done for so many. That was true up to about the 1980s. But by the time I went into practice, that had changed. It was an especially exciting time to be a neurologist because advances in research were producing medications that could dramatically improve a number of these conditions. The advances in medical treatment of migraine and MS had been life-changing for so many of my patients. Unfortunately, dementia was not one of those scientific success stories – at least, not then. The medicine chest for dementia was more of a time capsule, with little significant improvement since Dr. Alzheimer had first identified the disease nearly 100 years earlier.

Before the advent of acetylcholinesterase inhibitors like donepezil (Aricept), I was definitely, in clinical parlance, a lumper when it came to dementia. That is, I didn't worry about differentiating Alzheimer's disease from frontotemporal dementia (FTD), Lewy Body dementia, the dementia of Parkinson's disease, or vascular dementia. We had no medications to treat any of these types of dementia. All we knew was that most of these patients would progress to a state of complete loss of memory and total dependence on others for activities of daily living, and death would come in eight to ten years no matter what we did. I felt so helpless being unable to slow down the inexorable march of this disease.

The availability of donepezil in 1996 was a real turning point for me and others in the field, because it changed the way we could view dementia and the potential benefits of medication. An earlier acetylcholinesterase inhibitor (tacrine) had been approved in 1993, but it was so toxic to the liver that it was rarely used. Donepezil and two similar drugs released later (rivastigmine and galantamine) were much safer. These drugs increase the concentration of the neurotransmitter acetylcholine in memory circuits in the brain that are damaged by Alzheimer's disease. I started using donepezil in my patients with Alzheimer's, and often it helped, especially in those with mild to moderate memory impairment. Occasionally, the improvement was dramatic. Some people had no response at all, and others couldn't tolerate the common gastrointestinal side effects of cramping and diarrhea. Sometimes patients would be able to tolerate one of these drugs better than another, but they were all about equally effective. A fourth drug, memantine (Namenda) was approved in 2003. It works on a different pathway in the brain by blocking the so-called NMDA receptor for the excitatory neurotransmitter glutamate. It is not clear how this improves symptoms of Alzheimer's disease, but it can have a modest effect, especially when combined with other drugs.

It's important to emphasize that these drugs are not a cure for Alzheimer's disease. At best, they improve memory and other cognitive skills to the level they were one or two years before. The drugs have no effect on the spread of the plaques or tangles that lead to death of nerve cells. Cognition continues to worsen, but it does so from an improved level, buying some extra time.

The advent of an effective treatment for the symptoms of Alzheimer's disease – even if it couldn't resolve the cause – highlighted the need for an accurate diagnosis of the specific type of dementia a patient might have. Until this point, I had been a lumper. I treated all dementias the same – which is to say I didn't treat them at all because there was no treatment. Donepezil, rivastigmine, galantamine and memantine were at least partially effective for Alzheimer's disease. The first three also improved cognitive performance in Lewy Body dementia and the dementia of Parkinson's disease. However, they had no benefit for vascular dementia, and they could actually worsen the symptoms of frontotemporal dementia.

Like most neurologists, I had to hone my skills at differentiating the dementias based on the way symptoms presented case by case in the patients who came through the door. CT and MRI scans could help rule out mimics of dementia like brain tumors, subdural hematomas and normal-pressure hydrocephalus, but PET scans and spinal taps for biomarkers were not generally available until relatively recently. In general, Alzheimer's disease begins with memory problems as the earliest symptom. The hallmark of Lewy Body dementia is very early visual hallucinations, long before cognitive impairment starts. Parkinsonian features can occur later. The dementia of Parkinson's disease is usually straightforward because the tremors, rigid muscles, and gait disorders characteristic of Parkinson's precede the cognitive impairment. Frontotemporal dementia usually begins with behavioral issues before clear cognitive impairment, and it classically starts at an earlier age. Vascular dementia can mimic all of the other types and can be difficult to distinguish on the basis of symptoms and signs only. To make things more confusing, there is often overlap, with more than one type of dementia occurring in the same person. For the first time, I had to switch from lumping all the dementias together and start being a splitter – doing my best to make an accurate diagnosis of the type of dementia.

Adding to the diagnostic confusion was the occasional patient who would ultimately turn out to have Alzheimer's, but would present initially with another neurological problem and have no apparent cognitive impairment. I recall a woman in her late seventies who had started having spells of inattention and confusion that were suggestive of complex partial seizures, a focal epilepsy arising from the temporal or frontal lobes. The most common cause of new-onset seizures from middle age on is a stroke, but her MRI looked normal for age. There were no strokes, tumors or other focal lesions that might be expected to cause seizures. A normal MRI is not uncommon with new epilepsy, and it is reassuring. Her EEG showed intermittent abnormal electrical activity in her left temporal lobe which confirmed my suspicion of complex partial seizures. She responded well to a low dose of an anti-epileptic medication. The spells stopped entirely. However, about a year later, she started to develop cognitive impairment that within a few years was clearly due to Alzheimer's disease. Seizures are seven times more likely to occur in people with Alzheimer's disease than in those people of the same age who do not have dementia [1]. Although the seizures may develop in the late stages of the disease as a result of brain degeneration and scarring, they can also occur in the early stages, even before the beginning of noticeable cognitive impairment. They tend to be more common in those with an earlier onset of cognitive impairment, and are especially common in those with hereditary causes of Alzheimer's [2].

Another patient who was in her sixties was referred to me because of problems with her vision that her eye doctor felt were neurological in origin. Her neurological exam was completely normal except for a homonymous hemianopsia: she had impaired vision in the right visual fields of both eyes. This is classically seen in a stroke or tumor in the visual areas of the occipital or parietal lobe, but her MRI scan was normal. I was puzzled and saw her again in six months. Her vision was now impaired in both visual fields, and now she was starting to have some mild cognitive impairment. A repeat MRI scan still showed no stroke or tumor, but there was now some subtle atrophy in the occipital and parietal lobes of the brain. I referred her to a dementia expert who confirmed that she had poster-ior cortical atrophy, a rare variant of Alzheimer's disease in which the pathological hallmarks of amyloid plaques and neurofibrillary tangles are found first in the posterior parts of the brain, rather than in the frontal and temporal lobes. It typically has an earlier onset than Alzheimer's, usually in the fifties or sixties [3]. This was the only case of this disorder that I ever encountered.

As we've already seen, olfactory impairment occurs very early in Alzheimer's disease. Although virtually all people with Alzheimer's have some degree of loss of the ability to smell when tested, most are not aware of it. I became aware of my olfactory impairment at least six or seven years before any hint of cognitive impairment. I probably would not have noticed the decreased ability to smell had I not experienced the striking phantosmias, the illusory odors that weren't really there. In the last year I was in practice, I saw a man in his early sixties who was having in-trusive odors not associated with a true olfactory stimulus. They were always the same, and they were not unpleas-ant. They were brief in duration and, as such, I thought they were more consistent with olfactory seizures rather than phantosmias. He also had no symptoms of cognitive impairment, and cognitive testing was normal. His brain MRI was normal. Olfactory testing demonstrated minimal impairment. An EEG showed some abnormal sharp waves coming from the temporal lobe, a non-specific finding that would be consistent with seizures but also might be seen in Alzheimer's patients who did not have overt seizures. I tried him on an anti-epileptic medication, but there was no improvement in the frequency or duration of the intrusive smells. Within six months, he was starting to have noticeable cognitive impairment, and he almost certainly had early-stage Alzheimer's disease. Phantosmias, to my knowledge, have not been reported in association with Alzheimer's disease. However, after publication in *JAMA Neurology* in 2019 of my paper that included a description of my phantosmias, four people with, or at risk for, Alzheimer's contacted me by email to say that they too have experienced this phenomenon.

Now we are starting to learn that what we call Alzheimer's disease, based on clinically defined criteria and the specific neuropathological findings of amyloid plaques and tau-containing neurofibrillary tangles, may be more of a syndrome – a group of individual diseases, each with distinct genetic, anatomic and biochemical associations, and possibly different treatments. For example, Alzheimer's disease associated with the APOE-4 gene has some subtle – and, perhaps, not so subtle – differences from Alzheimer's disease in those without APOE-4. APOE-4 carriers have an increased incidence of ARIA during anti-amyloid drug trials [4], and this has been suggested to possibly result in a more robust response [5]. In another recent study, APOE-4 has been shown to have a deleterious effect on the mitochondria in the brain that is independent of amyloid and results in shrinkage and loss of neurons [6]. Then there is the extraordinary case of the Columbian woman with a presenilin 1 gene mutation that usually results in early-onset Alzheimer's and death before age 50. She lived until age 77 despite widespread amyloidosis in her brain by PET scan and only very mild cognitive impairment because she had the very rare occurrence of two copies of the APOE-3 Christchurch mutation, a genetic combination that seems to have protected her from the effects of amyloid [7].

This illustrates how much we have yet to learn about the interaction of genes, lifestyle and other factors that can impact the development of neurodegenerative diseases like Alzheimer's. Most of us have been lumpers, assuming that Alzheimer's is one disease, just as, thirty years ago, many of us would have considered that all dementias were pretty much alike. This may be one reason that clinical trials of possible disease-modifying drugs have been disappointing. In the early trials of anti-amyloid medications, the pool of research subjects was almost certainly contaminated by people with dementias other than Alzheimer's disease, making it harder to show possible effectiveness against Alzheimer's pathology. In current trials of Alzheimer's drugs, amyloid PET scans are required so that all subjects are known to have Alzheimer's pathology. This should increase the odds of success. But it may get more complicated. There is some evidence that APOE-4 carriers may respond differently to a disease-modifying drug than non-carriers, even though they all have positive amyloid PET scans and clinically fit the diagnosis of "Alzheimer's disease." What is the difference between APOE-4 carriers and non-carriers? Do they actually have the same disease? We don't really know. There are undoubtedly other genetic and biochemical variants that result in what we have been calling Alzheimer's disease, but which will require their own targeted therapies. We still have a lot to learn.

In their book *Brain Fables: The Hidden History of Neurodegenerative Diseases and a Blueprint to Conquer Them*, authors Alberto Espay, Professor of Neurology at the University of Cincinnati, and Parkinson's patient advocate Benjamin Stecher argue that this is the case for all the neurodegenerative diseases:

> *"Parkinson's" and "Alzheimer's" are too broad to be tackled. They are, biologically speaking, fictional constructs. The blueprint for conquering these diseases start[s] by studying the*

many pathways where normal aging can detour into abnormal aging in different individuals – even with the "same disease." We must keep our focus on small but achievable targets, regardless of whether they fall under "Parkinson's," "Alzheimer's," or any other man-made label. [8]

The Holy Grail of Alzheimer's disease investigation now is the search for a treatment that can halt the underlying disease process, a so-called disease-modifying intervention. So far, nothing has proved effective in clinical trials (with one possible exception), but there has been a lot of progress in understanding what happens in the brain during the disease, and a number of ways of intervening are being actively pursued. One reason that clinical trials have so far failed is that, by the time there has been significant memory impairment, a lot of damage has been done that may not be reversible. This realization has focused more recent trials on treating subjects in the earliest stages of the disease, sometimes even before there has been any cognitive impairment, and, not surprisingly, these subjects are hard to identify and recruit for studies. The shift in thinking about pre-symptomatic Alzheimer's disease, the ten or twenty years before cognitive impairment begins, is not without controversy. For one thing, not everyone who tests positive for brain amyloid will go on to develop Alzheimer's. There are those elderly people with positive amyloid scans who are cognitively normal for their age [9]. Not everyone with amyloid in the brain will develop Alzheimer's disease before they die. It is likely that the precision of preclinical diagnosis, finding markers before cognitive impairment starts, might be improved by using more than one biomarker, perhaps both amyloid PET and tau PET scans, or something new that has yet to be discovered. Blood tests for both beta-amyloid and tau appear to be on the horizon, and when these become available it should be much easier to make an early diagnosis of Alzheimer's [10].

It is also possible that one type of medication will not work for all subtypes of Alzheimer's disease. Perhaps different approaches will be needed for APOE-4 carriers and non-carriers, for those with other genetic risks. It's going to be complicated, but understanding the complexity will inform the search for new potential cures. In the meantime, on an individual level, those of us at risk need to adopt the lifestyle choices that have been shown to slow the progression of the disease.

Chapter-references

1   Irizarry MC, Jin S, He F, *et al*. Incidence of new-onset seizures in mild to moderate Alzheimer disease. *Archives of Neurology* 2012; 69:368–372; https://doi .org/10.1001/archneurol.2011.830 (public access version available at www.ncbi.nlm.nih.gov/pmc/ articles/PMC3622046).

2   Vossel KA, Beagle AJ, Rabinovici G, *et al*. Seizures and epileptiform activity in the early stages of Alzheimer disease. *JAMA Neurology* 2013; 70:1158–1166; https:// doi.org/10.1001/jamaneurol.2013.136 (public access version available at www.ncbi.nlm.nih.gov/pmc/ articles/PMC4013391).

3   Crutch SJ, Lehmann M, Schott JM, *et al*. Posterior cortical atrophy. *Lancet Neurology* 2012; 11:170–178; https://doi.org/10.1016/S1474-4422(11)70289-7 (public access version available at www.ncbi.nlm.nih.gov/ pmc/articles/PMC3740271).

4   Salloway S, Sperling R, Fox NC, *et al*. Two phase 3 trials of bapineuzumab in mild-to-moderate Alzheimer's disease. *New England Journal of Medicine* 2014; 370:322– 333 (public access version available at www.ncbi.nlm .nih.gov/pmc/articles/PMC4159618).

5   Knopman, DS. Sifting through a failed Alzheimer trial: what biomarkers tell us about what happened.

Neurology 2018; 90:447–448; https://doi.org/10.1212/
WNL.0000000000005073.

6 Yin J, Reiman EM, Beach TG, *et al*. Effect of ApoE
   isoforms on mitochondria in Alzheimer disease.
   Neurology 2020; 94:e2404–e2411; https://doi.org/
   10.1212/WNL.0000000000009582.

7 Arboleda-Velasquez, JF, Lopera F, O'Hare M, *et al*.
   Resistance to autosomal dominant Alzheimer's
   disease in an *APOE3* Christchurch homozygote: a case
   report. *Nature Medicine* 2019; 25:1680–1683; https://doi
   .org/10.1038/s41591-019–0611-3 (public access version
   available at www.ncbi.nlm.nih.gov/pmc/articles/
   PMC6898984).

8 Espay A, Stecher B. *Brain Fables: The Hidden History of
   Neurodegenerative Diseases and a Blueprint to Conquer
   Them*. Cambridge University Press, 2020.

9 Chételat G, La Joie R, Villain N, *et al*. Amyloid imaging
   in cognitively normal individuals, at-risk populations
   and preclinical Alzheimer's disease. *NeuroImage:
   Clinical*, 2013; 2:356–365; https://doi.org/10.1016/j
   .nicl.2013.02.006 (public access version available at
   www.ncbi.nlm.nih.gov/pmc/articles/PMC3777672).

10 Palmqvist S, Janelidze S, Quiroz YT, *et al*.
   Discriminative accuracy of plasma phospho-tau217
   for Alzheimer disease vs other neurodegenerative
   disorders. JAMA 2020; 324:772–781; https://doi
   .org/10.1001/jama.2020.12134 (public access version
   available at https://jamanetwork.com/journals/jama/
   fullarticle/2768841).

21 A MEANINGFUL OUTCOME

Memory loss is the familiar headliner, but one of the most insidious symptoms of Alzheimer's disease is apathy. Not as in a casual indifference or uncaring attitude that might change if you understood more about a thing at hand. For someone with Alzheimer's, apathy is biological, intrinsic to the disease as it affects the brain's executive function and diminishes motivation and the capacity to make plans and follow through. It's as if your brain has gotten the kit for caring and empathy, but with no way to assemble it – the anatomical structures and mechanisms in the brain that would do that are damaged. Apathy is considered the most common neuropsychiatric symptom of those with Alzheimer's. A recent meta-analysis covering twenty-five studies showed a prevalence of apathy in Alzheimer's ranging from 19 percent to 88 percent – quite a range, but with an overall mean or mid-point prevalence of 49 percent, meaning that apathy was a clinical issue for at least half those in the overall participant population [1].

The psychological toll only adds to that and includes others, such as caregivers, for whom feelings of helplessness and hopelessness can become so formidable. The meta-analysis also pointed out that the notably wide range of prevalence reflected the lack of more discerning tools to identify differences in the severity of the disease, and of the apathy itself. In other words, more research is needed into this most common symptom, which has such a profound effect on those with Alzheimer's, their families and caregivers.

It is tempting to give up and say, "There is nothing I can do, there is no hope, why bother?" I fight against my apathy all the time, and I know that the fight is worth it. I feel so much better when I can take action and feel that I am in charge, not Alzheimer's. But for those of us with the disease, even its earliest stages, it's daunting to get your head around the idea of taking charge against a disease that is slowly destroying your brain.

Apathy on a societal scale is a problem, too, with consequences on a larger scale, affecting funding for research, medical, healthcare and community initiatives that are so sorely needed. As a society, how can we take charge of a disease that afflicts nearly 6 million Americans today, is estimated to more than double that by 2050, and threatens so many millions more, globally?

We can take meaningful steps to counter apathy, personally and collectively. Here is how:

Take it personally. To start, those of us with Alzheimer's or increased risk of it can embrace the lifestyle choices that have been shown to slow the progression of the disease. These include daily aerobic exercise, following a heart-healthy diet such as the Mediterranean or MIND diets, staying intellectually and socially engaged, and getting adequate, restorative sleep. Don't wait. These lifestyle choices are most effective if started at the earliest stages of the disease, even before there are cognitive symptoms, perhaps as early as age 40 for people who are at higher risk. If you know someone, perhaps a parent or other older relative, either who is at risk or whose behavior has worried you, advocate for a visit to their physician to rule out whatever they can and focus on the actual source of the problem.

Learn about Alzheimer's. For patients and their families, as well as healthcare providers, the Alzheimer's

Association is a wonderful source of information, support and programs including a 24/7 telephone support line.[1] The Alzheimer's Association is also the largest non-governmental source of funding for dementia research in the world. In the UK, the Alzheimer's Society provides many of the same services.[2]

Volunteer. As a neurologist and former research scientist, I feel certain that effective, disease-modifying medications – drugs that will slow progression or even cure Alzheimer's disease if started early enough, and perhaps even prevent the disease altogether in people at risk who have not yet developed symptoms – can be discovered in time for my children's generation, if not for mine. Eventually, we will discover ways of treating the more advanced disease, but learning how to regenerate or replace dead and dying nerve cells is a challenge that may take many years. Finding a cure for Alzheimer's disease will take many, many volunteer research subjects, probably hundreds of thousands. Most needed will be those who are at risk because of a family history of dementia or have known genetic markers but who don't yet have cognitive impairment. Having parents or a sibling with Alzheimer's, especially if combined with pre-cognitive symptoms like progressive olfactory loss or smelling illusory odors, would increase the chances that one might be a good candidate for a drug study aimed at early-stage disease. Being a part of the aducanumab study was an extraordinary experience for me. It provided structure to my life for two years. I made new friends among the doctors, nurses and other staff at the research center. It was intellectually stimulating. Despite the adverse side effects I experienced, I think I have improved cognitively since the trial. Most importantly, I feel that I have made a contribution to finding a cure, and for

[1]   Alzheimer's Association website: www.alz.org.
[2]   Alzheimer's Society (UK) website: www.alzheimers.org.uk.

that I am both happy and proud. To find information about clinical trials near you, go to the Alzheimer's Association TrialMatch webpage[3] or the NIH website clinicaltrials.gov.

Support science and the work to be done. That's where the answers will be found. The cost of this needed research is high, but it pales in comparison to the cost to society of Alzheimer's, in the financial cost of lost productivity and long-term care as well as the human cost to Alzheimer's patients and their caregivers. Society needs to take responsibility for a larger share of the cost of this research, rather than relying too much on the pharmaceutical industry. The drug companies have been essential partners in the search for a cure for Alzheimer's, but they are ultimately driven by the potential for profit. Their costs to conduct large clinical trials are enormous, and when the trials appear to have failed in achieving the primary endpoint for success, the companies usually drop further investigation to minimize their losses. For example, interest in anti-amyloid monoclonal antibodies has waned after multiple trial failures. But subgroup analysis of these trials tends to show that there may be some benefit at higher doses, in those subjects who have ARIA, and in those who carry the APOE-4 gene.

Teasing out those potential benefits will be expensive, and, so far, the drug companies don't seem very interested in pursuing those leads. There are several studies that suggest that generically available medications for inflammation and diabetes might have some benefit in treating Alzheimer's disease, but no drug company is likely to take on the cost of large clinical trials because there would be limited profit potential from a drug that has no patent protection. One major company recently failed to disclose its own research suggesting that one of its drugs for

---

[3] TrialMatch website: www.alz.org/alzheimers-dementia/research_progress/clinical-trials/about-clinical-trials.

rheumatoid arthritis might provide some modest protection against getting Alzheimer's. The rationale for burying the study appeared to be based on the limited time left for patent protection of this drug, so there would be no way to make money from it [2].

I don't particularly fault the pharmaceutical industry. Despite the TV ads, these companies are not in the business of altruism. They are in the business of creating profit for their investors. We shouldn't rely on the industry to fund all Alzheimer's disease research. Substantial funding must come from government agencies and private foundations like the Alzheimer's Association.

But what we really need is a change in the research model. Instead of competition between companies, academic scientists and even countries to be the first to succeed in finding new cures, new patents and huge financial returns, there needs to be a common, coordinated battle, sharing information, research models, and promising leads on drugs or other interventions that might be effective. I think there is a glimmer of hope for more cooperation between drug companies, academic scientists and government agencies going forward. The response to the Covid-19 pandemic has been a remarkable model of data sharing and cooperative studies involving many stakeholders. My hope is that the world will soon wake up to the explicit threat of the growing pandemic of Alzheimer's disease and attack it with the same determination, ingenuity and cooperation we are seeing now in response to Covid-19.

The passion is certainly there in the science community, and it needs to be matched elsewhere. Consider Allen Roses, a maverick Alzheimer's researcher at Duke University when he discovered the connection between APOE-4 and Alzheimer's disease in the early 1990s [3]. His findings were initially controversial. The possible connection with a gene connected to lipid transport did not fit into the paradigm of how Alzheimer's was thought to work. According to his obituary in the *New York Times* [4], some of his research had to be financed by a personal loan secured by his house. Today, the relationship between APOE-4 and risk for Alzheimer's is fully accepted, while not yet completely understood. The contributions of dedicated scientists and others in the field are ongoing. Funding needs to catch up.

Be an everyday advocate. There is still much misunderstanding and stigma associated with Alzheimer's disease. I talk about my experiences and what I have learned to anyone who will listen: medical students, physicians, Alzheimer's researchers, people with dementia, families of people with dementia, my own friends and family, and the media. The benefits of research go beyond the search for a cure. Responsible, evidence-based conversation about any disease or medical condition raises awareness, challenges myths and stigmas that hurt people, and sometimes can help sufferers themselves understand what's happening to them and why, which can be hugely beneficial. The more we talk about it, and the sooner we do, the sooner the barriers will start to fall, and better understanding, care and treatment will follow.

For example, early in my private-practice years, I became interested in the connection between changes in brain blood flow and symptoms of panic attacks. In my previous work as a research scientist, I had studied the neuroendocrinology of stress, including the role of blood flow and its effect on the mechanisms in the brain involved in anxiety and panic attacks. I did training in neurovascular sonology, the use of ultrasound waves to measure blood flow velocities in the carotid arteries of the neck and large arteries of the brain. This became a significant part of my practice. Initially, it was used mainly for patients at risk for stroke or who had already had a stroke or TIAs (transient ischemic attacks). These transcranial Doppler ultrasound techniques were helpful in identifying regions of significant arterial narrowing or stenosis, both in the carotid arteries and in the intracranial arteries, including the anterior, middle and posterior cerebral arteries as well as the vertebral and basilar arteries.

I found an unexpected use for these ultrasound techniques when I started to see a number of patients with panic disorder, who frequently suffered panic attacks. These patients had been referred because they were having symptoms suggestive of a neurological disorder. Panic attacks are defined as unexpected episodes consisting of four or more common symptoms for which there is no determined medical cause, such as heart rhythm problems, TIAs or stroke, epileptic seizures or medication side effects. These include: shortness of breath; palpitations or accelerated heart rate; feeling dizzy, lightheaded or faint; sweating; trembling or shaking; feeling of choking; chest pain; nausea or abdominal distress; feelings of unreality or depersonalization; fear of losing control or going crazy; fear of dying; numbness and tingling; chills or hot flushes. Any one of those is plenty to struggle with – and many patients experience most or all of them.

In 1990, I was asked to evaluate a 44-year-old man whose problems had started when he began to have unexplained episodes of passing out as a teen. The spells resolved when he was a young adult but returned at age 40, along with severe anxiety. At the peak, he would pass out five to seven times per day. He had already had extensive cardiac and neurological evaluations that were all normal. He also had more typical panic attacks daily, but no one felt comfortable attributing his spells of passing out to panic attacks. I tested him with the transcranial Doppler and was shocked to find that, during hyperventilation, the blood flow in his basilar artery, the major blood supply to the brain stem and back of the brain, decreased by over 80 percent.

Everybody has a decrease in blood flow to the brain during hyperventilation. That's why we feel dizzy and our hands tingle when we over-breathe. This decrease in blood flow is caused by a drop of carbon dioxide levels in the blood caused by hyperventilation. Normal people have on average only a 35 to 40 percent decrease in this blood flow when they over-breathe. This patient's reduction in blood flow when he hyperventilated was so extreme that it caused him to lose consciousness. This made me wonder whether the intracranial arteries of people with panic disorder might be more sensitive to the changes in carbon dioxide in blood that occur during hyperventilation, and might therefore have a greater decrease in blood flow than those of people who don't have panic disorder. I did a small study comparing nine patients with panic disorder to nine normal controls. The patients with panic disorder had an average 62 percent reduction in basilar artery blood flow during hyperventilation, compared to 36 percent in control subjects. In other words, when people with panic disorder over-breathe, they have a greater reduction of blood flow to the brain than do people without panic disorder. I think this is probably the physiological mechanism behind at least some of the symptoms that occur during a panic attack, such as dizziness, shortness of breath, and numbness and tingling [5].

People who suffer from panic attacks often have trouble getting proper treatment. Frequently they are concerned that there is something seriously physically wrong – a stroke or heart attack, for instance – and these concerns are reasonable since symptoms of a panic attack often include an irregular heart rate. A stroke or even a seizure can cause similar symptoms. Once a physician has ruled out these conditions, it is not uncommon for the patient to be told that "It's all in your head," without being provided with further explanation or treatment. In patients who truly have panic attacks, I found it to be very helpful to demonstrate to them in real time the marked reduction in blood flow to the brain that they can see on the screen of the transcranial Doppler machine as they experience their typical symptoms. It's like a light has gone on as they suddenly understand the cause of their symptoms, and it helps them feel more comfortable about following up with appropriate treatment, whether it be as simple as breathing into a paper bag during an attack to keep the carbon dioxide level from falling in the blood, starting one of the medications available for panic disorder, or undergoing other psychotherapeutic treatment.

My hope is that, as we discover and communicate to the public more about the earliest stages of Alzheimer's, long before symptoms begin to emerge, we can normalize the conversation and help more people to seek out the professional guidance, and sometimes the medication, that might help them the most. The seemingly quirky olfactory issues that came up for me are a good example. As research now confirms, almost all people with Alzheimer's disease have at least some impairment of the ability to smell, but over 90 percent of them are unaware of this until tested. Since they tend to be tested only when other symptoms of cognitive decline or changes in behavior have begun to emerge, they are typically in the later stages of the disease, long after the overlooked olfactory symptom might have been noted for follow-up, perhaps allowing for treatment that might have slowed the progression of the disease. By then it's too late.

I say this with certainty. I may not recall the books I read a month ago, but my memory of my patients' experience earlier in my career, and now my own – my memory for the clinical narrative of Alzheimer's disease for the past thirty years – is undiminished, and that past must inform the present.

Neuroscience has so many ways to define and describe the mechanisms of memory and the way that Alzheimer's corrupts the connections and threatens to disable the system. But, in purely human terms, what's at stake in memory loss is our fundamental sense of self: who we are, what we know and feel and believe, and how we belong and live in the world. Memory and memories create us. They define our self to ourselves and one another in the most profound ways. When we talk about buying time with earlier diagnosis and treatment, that's what we're talking about. There is no time to lose.

Chapter-references

1   Nobis L, Husain M. Apathy in Alzheimer's disease. *Current Opinion in Behavioral Sciences* 2018; 22:7–13; https://doi.org/10.1016/j.cobeha.2017.12.007 (public access version available at www.ncbi.nlm.nih.gov/pmc/articles/PMC6095925).

2   Rowland, C. Pfizer had clues its blockbuster drug could prevent Alzheimer's. Why didn't it tell the world? *The Washington Post* June 4, 2019; www .washingtonpost.com/business/economy/pfizer-had-clues-its-blockbuster-drug-could-prevent-alzheimers-why-didnt-it-tell-the-world/2019/06/04/9092e08a-7a61-11e9-8bb7-0fc796cf2ec0_story.html.

3   Roses AD. Apolipoprotein E alleles as risk factors in Alzheimer's disease. *Annual Review of Medicine* 1996; 47:387–400; https://doi.org/10.1146/annurev.med .47.1.387.

4   Allen Roses, who upset common wisdom on cause of Alzheimer's, dies at 73. *New York Times* October 5, 2016; www.nytimes.com/2016/10/06/science/allen-roses-who-upset-common-wisdom-on-cause-of-alzheimers-dies-at-73.html.

5   Gibbs DM. Hyperventilation-induced cerebral ischemia in panic disorder and effect of nimodipine. *American Journal of Psychiatry* 1992; 149(11):1589–1591; https://doi.org/10.1176/ajp.149.11.1589.

EPILOGUE: THE WRITING LIFE

I was up by 5:30 a.m., to give myself plenty of time for an unhurried arrival at the 7:30 a.m. breakfast meeting scheduled at a downtown Portland restaurant. I had been there several times before, most recently about three months earlier. As I got ready to leave the house, already a little behind schedule, I discovered that my cell phone had not charged overnight and was now completely dead. I plugged it in to charge and left the house.

The streetcar took me to the Portland State University stop, and I had a pretty good mental image of where the restaurant was, although I couldn't exactly remember whether it was on S.W. Fourth or Sixth Street. I looked on Sixth for a few blocks. Nothing looked familiar. I walked over to Fourth Street. It looked even less familiar. I was now late for my appointment. I had no phone to call and say I was late. I couldn't even check the address of the restaurant. I started to panic. I ran back to Sixth and looked a few more blocks from where I had looked before. Still nothing familiar. I ran back to Fourth. Still nothing. I was now ten minutes late – highly uncharacteristic for me, which only made me all the more frustrated. Finally, I stopped a couple walking on Fourth Street and asked if they knew where the restaurant was. The guy checked his smartphone and gave me the address. It turned out that I was also off on the cross street by about four blocks, and thus I was six blocks from the restaurant. I ran all the way there. Just as I reached the place, my digital watch activity tracker dinged and messaged me that it was now tracking my "outdoor run." I shut it off dismissively and met my companions. I was flustered and embarrassed. Only later did I discover that the activity tracker had given me credit for a 0.47-mile run. All to the good as final tallies go, but it sure wasn't what I'd expected.

I could say the same about writing this book. When I wrote the brief personal essay that appeared in *JAMA Neurology* in spring of 2019, it was to share, as a retired neurologist writing to other neurologists, my experiences as a patient with Alzheimer's disease. I wanted to encourage them to seek more actively to detect and treat Alzheimer's in its earliest stages, when a patient's lifestyle choices have the greatest chance to alter the neurodegenerative course of the disease – a chance to slow cognitive impairment, and extend the largely pre-symptomatic stage by ten to twenty years. I began writing this book as an expansion of that piece, still focused on pressing for change in the medical profession, especially among those physicians on the front lines with patients who might benefit.

Along the way, in the process of putting my memories on the page, I discovered there was more to it than I had anticipated. Writing at length could be challenging, especially when my Alzheimer's would trip me up occasionally over some of the simplest things. When ideas come to me while I'm doing something else (walking with Jack, making coffee, talking about a book with Lois), I have to be sure to make a written note of it immediately. I mean I have to stop what I am doing and jot down the note or the thought will be lost. Mental notes just aren't as reliable as they once were. My early dementia affects my verbal memory, so it is not uncommon for me to have trouble coming up with a word I want. It's easy for me to lose the thread that I want to write about. I have to avoid distractions. I can't listen to music and I have to self-isolate. I usually write at my desk in the study, sometimes with the door

shut. Otherwise I can't concentrate enough to get anything down on the page. Perhaps surprisingly, sometimes
I do get on a roll and write for quite a while, each sentence
informing the next.

I was somewhat surprised to discover that when I focus on a particular memory – family, friends, colleagues
or, many times, patients and places – even from the distant past, I often remember more than I can possibly use.
I filled pages with memories from my years as a research
scientist before I finished my training in neurology and became a neurologist. All told, I had published thirty-five scientific and medical papers, on twenty-two of which I was
the first author – and often the only author, meaning that
I actually wrote the paper. I'd always enjoyed the scientific
writing and it is an unexpected pleasure now to be able to
revisit that part of my life.

Other memories remained vivid as well – all of them colorful side streets on the way to a finished manuscript. It is
a gift to spend unhurried time in those thoughts, about my
childhood, life with Lois and the kids, cherished friends
and a challenging, satisfying career. The work of writing
is also a welcome taskmaster, an obligation of choice. Lois
and I spend many weekends at the Oregon coast, and, between long walks and slow sunsets, the writing gives me
some useful structure and purpose.

Most writers have a favored time of day for it, the time
when they feel most creative or productive. I always
thought that morning was my best time to write, and I still
do write nearly every morning for a couple of hours after
walking Jack. Recently, as I've felt some pressure to get
this manuscript completed, I've started working at night,
too. That has worked very well, despite the occasional beer
or wine with dinner. I think it is because there are fewer
distractions. Jack usually settles down in the evening until
his bedtime at 10, so I feed him a snack then and we both
go to bed.

I usually write on my laptop; my typing is no worse for wear. I often keep my iPad open to catch texts and emails because my laptop screen is too small to comfortably keep more than one window open at a time. Once I minimize or close a window, the content is gone from my brain. Sometimes I make written notes on a pad of paper using a ballpoint pen or pencil – whatever is handy. I've been running through the ballpoints, so a pencil has to do at times. But let's face it: the most important writing instrument is your brain.

Writing involves interaction of many centers and pathways throughout the brain, and all of these need to be functioning properly for fluent writing to occur. These areas include those for language processing in the left frontal and temporal lobes, spelling (orthographic) centers in the parietal lobe, visual perception in the occipital and parietal lobes, and motor control of handwriting in the frontal lobe motor cortex. Impairment of writing, including misspellings, omitted letters, and writing the wrong word, can start early in some people with Alzheimer's disease. I've noted that I make far more spelling mistakes than I used to. Spellcheck usually takes care of these slips for me. Reading is somewhat less complicated, primarily involving the occipital and temporal lobes and the connecting fiber bundle called the inferior longitudinal fasciculus, which connects the visual centers in the occipital lobes with language processing centers in the left temporal lobe [1]. The loss of the ability to read is called alexia. When I was in the middle of the ARIA episode, I couldn't read (alexia) but I could still write. With the resolution of the brain edema from ARIA, my ability to read returned essentially to normal, and my ability to write remains only minimally impaired by the Alzheimer's.

The irony of my brain's changing capacity to remember some things past with such clarity, and yet to forget others, is not lost on me. Very early in my career, I studied the neuro-muscular pharmacology of a swallowing muscle in the sea slug, *Aplysia californica*, which resulted in co-authorship of my first research paper, published in 1977 [2]. How can it be that my memory of that study is more accessible to me than the location of the restaurant that eluded me so recently?

The one constant I do not lose sight of is my purpose in writing this book: to share what I have learned so it can help others. The pathological changes of Alzheimer's disease begin in the brain up to twenty years before the onset of cognitive impairment. There now is overwhelming evidence that simple lifestyle changes started during this period can markedly slow the progression of Alzheimer's. I believe that a cure will eventually be found, but until that happens we need to focus on these early stages, before memory is lost, and start fighting the battle before it is too late. Whatever it takes to get that word out, I'm on it.

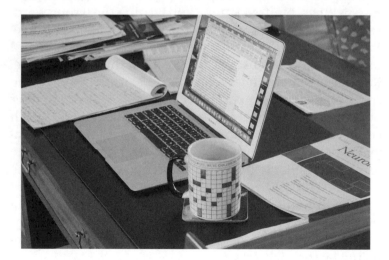

My desk while writing this book.

Chapter-references

1   Wandell BA, Le RK. Diagnosing the neural circuitry of reading. *Neuron* 2017; 96:298–311; https://doi .org/10.1016/j.neuron.2017.08.007 (open access).
2   Taraskevich PS, Gibbs D, Schmued L, Orkand RK. Excitatory effects of cholinergic, adrenergic and glutaminergic agonists on a buccal muscle of Aplysia. *Developmental Neurobiology* 1977; 8:325–335; https://doi .org/10.1002/neu.480080405.

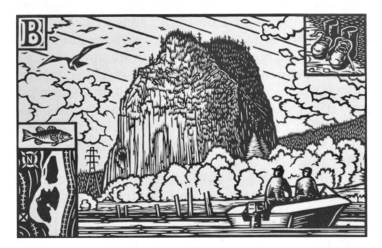

"B is for Beacon," block print by Dennis Cunningham (www.denniscunningham.net). Used by permission.

EPILOGUE: THE WRITING LIFE, ACT II

July 2022

I never imagined that my weekly ritual of sorting pills by the bathroom sink would someday draw an audience. Much less a documentary filmmaker and crew with cameras, lights, and sound equipment perched on the counter for the best angle. It wasn't what I expected in this lifetime, but then I could say the same about writing this book.

When I penned the brief personal essay that appeared in *JAMA Neurology* in the winter of 2019, it was to share, as a retired neurologist writing to other neurologists, my experiences as a patient with Alzheimer's disease. I wanted to encourage them to seek more actively to detect and manage Alzheimer's in its earliest stages, when a patient's lifestyle choices have the greatest chance to alter the neurodegenerative course of the disease – a chance to extend the pre-symptomatic stage and slow the progression of cognitive impairment. I began writing this book as an expansion of that piece, still focused on pressing for change in the medical profession, especially among those physicians on the front lines with patients who might benefit.

Along the way, in the process of putting my memories on the page, I discovered there was more to it than I had anticipated. Writing at length could be challenging, especially when my Alzheimer's would trip me up occasionally over some of the simplest things. When ideas come to me while I'm doing something else (walking with Jack, making coffee, talking about a book with Lois), I have to be sure to make a written note of it immediately. Not just soon. I mean I have to stop what I am doing right then and jot down the note or the thought will be lost. Mental notes just don't work anymore.

My early-stage dementia affects my verbal memory, so it is not uncommon for me to have trouble coming up with a word I want. It's easy for me to lose the thread that I want to write about. I have to avoid distractions. I can't listen to music and I have to self-isolate. I usually write at my desk in the study, sometimes with the door shut. Otherwise I can't concentrate enough to get anything down on the page. Perhaps surprisingly, sometimes I do get on a roll and write for quite a while, each sentence guiding my mind to the next, uninterrupted by Alzheimer's spotty neurological lapses.

I've also learned a lot in this new writing relationship with my brain. I was somewhat surprised to discover that when I focus on a particular memory – family, friends, colleagues or, many times, patients and places – even from the distant past, I often remember more than I can possibly use. Early on, I filled pages and pages with memories from my years as a research scientist before I finished my training in neurology and became a neurologist. All told, I had published thirty-five scientific and medical papers, on twenty-two of which I was the first author – and often the only author, meaning that I actually wrote the paper. I'd always enjoyed the scientific writing and it is an unexpected pleasure now to be able to revisit that part of my life.

Other memories remained vivid as well, all of them colorful side streets on the way to a finished manuscript. It is a gift to spend unhurried time in those thoughts, about my childhood, life with Lois and the kids, cherished friends, and a challenging, satisfying career. The work of writing is also a welcome taskmaster, an obligation of choice. Lois and I spend many weekends at the Oregon coast, and, between long walks and slow sunsets, the writing gives me some useful structure and purpose.

Most writers have a favored time of day for it, the time when they feel most creative or productive. I always thought that morning was my best time to write, and I still do write nearly every morning for a couple of hours after walking Jack. The difference now, with Alzheimer's, is that the sweet spot for cognitive function is more pronounced, the onset of the slight fog more predictable, so it's not only writing that I aim to do in my brain's prime time. I try to schedule anything that requires my full attention for those hours. That wasn't particularly challenging as I was writing the book, but starting the month before the book was released April 2021, intense media attention changed all that.

In the year since *A Tattoo on My Brain* came out, I have done thirty interviews and talks about the book: thirteen podcasts, nine radio, five print, one TV, one webinar, and one keynote address. Zoom interviews, phone calls, news media in our living room or on walks through the woods – a veritable whirlwind. Starting out, I was incredibly stressed about doing the interviews, especially the live ones that wouldn't allow for editing out my glitches or incidental barks from my dog Jack. As time went on, I grew more comfortable with the process.

Most of the interviewers asked similar questions, so I grew more practiced with my responses – an encouraging sign of my brain's capacity to keep learning. It was a growing experience in other ways, too. Long something of an introvert, I shed my aversion to public attention and agreed to do the interviews because I wanted the book to be widely read and quickly get the message out: the time to recognize and manage Alzheimer's disease is in the early stages, even before cognitive impairment has begun. The reaction to media coverage was tremendous and moved the message faster and farther still. When an interview with Rita Rubin, a writer for *JAMA (Journal of the American Medical Association)*, was published, I was astounded at the response from other physicians [1]. More than 29,000 read the interview online, and many contacted me by email.

Participating in clinical trials continues to be a major part of my life. I frankly have lost count of all of the studies I have been in. I don't expect that any particular study will benefit me, but I know that I am contributing to the wealth of knowledge about Alzheimer's. I am helping to build that pyramid. As the knowledge base expands, we will get closer and closer to effective management of Alzheimer's, to place the last blocks at the top of the pyramid.

Despite the controversy last year over the FDA approval of aducanumab, the anti-amyloid monoclonal antibody that put me in the ICU with life-threatening brain swelling and bleeding, I think we have learned a lot from this drug. It may turn out to be an effective treatment for some people with Alzheimer's disease, perhaps those with very early disease and certain genetic characteristics, but we just don't know yet. We need more information to balance any possible benefit with the risk of adverse reactions. Many other drugs are being tested in trials. Some are being tested in the pre-symptomatic stages before cognitive impairment has started. More and more studies are looking at the role of lifestyle modifications in slowing the progression of Alzheimer's and reducing the risk of getting it. I look forward to opportunities ahead to participate in trials of new advances in scanning and other technologies. Who knows? Maybe they will shed more light on the causes of and possible treatments for Alzheimer's. It is an extremely exciting time in Alzheimer's research, but we have to be patient. We have to follow the science.

After six months in the media spotlight, I thought it was a wrap and settled into a rhythm of Alzheimer's advocacy on other fronts, family activity, travel, though much constricted by Covid-19, and writing. I launched a blog to share updates and my thoughts about Alzheimer's news, as well as entries from my personal journey, including

photography (https://tattooonmybrain.com/). It was exciting to learn new tech tricks and discover a new social
space through comments on my blog. All in all, my interview season, while a little stressful at times, was engaging
and intellectually stimulating. I missed that a little, but appreciated that I now had more time to get on with the rest
of my life. Then came the call that would change everything – again. And eventually lead to the film crew on my
bathroom counter.

Somehow someone in the film industry had come
across my book, and the next thing I knew *Tattoo* was in
the hands of a master documentary filmmaker and thus
another new chapter of this experience is unfolding. I am
beyond grateful, not only for this unexpected and extraordinary life experience, but for the way the film will succeed in reaching even more people, an audience at a scale
I could never have imagined.

I am also relieved that I wrote the book when I did. Early in the painstaking process of hammering out the book-
to-film details of the *Tattoo* project, everyone agreed to
fast-track the process because of, as one diplomatic person called it, my "health predicament." And at one point,
when the question arose about the possibility of a sequel,
I confess that I didn't have a lot of patience for it. All I
could think was, let's just get on with this – there will be
no sequel unless someone else writes it posthumously!
Fortunately, the fast track delivered the film crew to our
doorstep in a matter of days, and the rest has been a fascinating and fun experience.

Once the crew packed up and our lives settled back to
the familiar pace and content of a day, I happily resumed
writing my blog. I'm still writing and enjoying it, but I'm
acutely attuned to the neurological complexity of that
task. Writing involves interaction of many centers and
pathways throughout the brain, and all of these need to
be functioning properly for fluent writing to occur. These

areas include those for language processing in the left frontal and temporal lobes, spelling (orthographic) centers in the parietal lobe, visual perception in the occipital and parietal lobes, and motor control of handwriting in the frontal lobe motor cortex. Impairment of writing, including misspellings, omitted letters, and writing the wrong word, can start early in some people with Alzheimer's disease. I've noted that I make far more spelling mistakes than I used to. Spellcheck usually takes care of these slips for me.

As for other activities, reading is somewhat less challenging for me because it is somewhat less complicated for the brain. It primarily involves the occipital and temporal lobes, and the connecting fiber bundle called the inferior longitudinal fasciculus, which connects the visual centers in the occipital lobes with language processing centers in the left temporal lobe [2]. The loss of the ability to read is called alexia. When I was in the middle of the ARIA episode, I couldn't read (alexia), but I could still write. With the resolution of the brain edema from ARIA, my ability to read returned essentially to normal, and my ability to write remains only minimally impaired by the Alzheimer's.

As for memory, the irony of my brain's changing capacity to remember some things past with such clarity, and yet to forget others, is not lost on me. Very early in my career, I studied the neuro-muscular pharmacology of a swallowing muscle in the sea slug, *Aplysia californica*, which resulted in co-authorship of my first research paper, published in 1977 [3]. How can it be that my memory of that study is more accessible to me than the location of the restaurant that eluded me so recently?

Whatever course the Alzheimer's runs, however the mysteries of the brain and this disease may change my cognitive status, one constant I do not lose sight of is my purpose in writing this book: to share what I have learned so it can help others. You'll understand if I want to underscore this: the pathological changes of Alzheimer's disease begin in the brain up to twenty years before the onset of cognitive impairment. There continues to be overwhelming evidence that simple lifestyle changes started during this period can markedly slow the progression of Alzheimer's. I believe that a cure will eventually be found, but until that happens, we need to focus on these early stages, before memory is lost, and start fighting the battle before it is too late. Whatever it takes to get that word out, I'm on it. I consider every day a fresh opportunity to work with that intention – and to live life fully with my loving family and friends, and nature always my companion.

Last summer Fourth of July celebrations were mostly cancelled because of COVID concerns. Interacting with family was more likely to be by Zoom than in person. That's why it felt so special this year to gather with family on the Oregon Coast for the holiday weekend. Two of our three children and their husbands, two grandchildren, and two dogs crowded in together to celebrate. Our two-year-old granddaughter was too young to stay up late enough to watch the fireworks launched less than a mile away (amazingly she slept through them), but her five-year-old sister stayed up to watch the display. It was her very first time to see fireworks, and she was absolutely thrilled. Watching her excitement brought tears to my eyes, and reminded me what we have missed so much this last year: being together to share the joy of families. And there was more in store – another grandchild to celebrate!

I take every opportunity to trek up Beacon Rock and was delighted when the film crew asked to go, too. To be able share special places new to someone else is a wonderful thing. And then there are the old places that grow all the more special over time with old friends. Last August, John, Henry and I made our annual sailing trip around the San Juans. Even though we have been sailing these waters each summer for over twenty years, we always see something new, like the huge Douglas fir growing out of the remains of its predecessors on Jones Island, or the six-mile round trip hike to the lighthouse on Stuart Island. It's all good. But the best part is reuniting with old friends, now aging into our seventies, sharing stories, giving updates on children and grandchildren, playing hearts badly after dinner and a glass or two of wine, and generally having one heck of a wonderful time. Getting out on a boat, catching up with friends, and hiking on mountain trails, what better emotional therapy can there be?

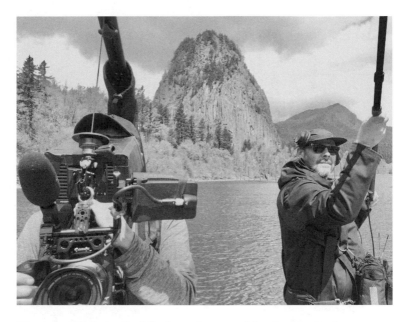

Film crew filming me while I am photographing Beacon Rock.

Chapter-references

1   Rubin R. Neurologist faces his Alzheimer diagnosis determined to lessen stigma surrounding the disease. *JAMA* 2021; 325:1926–1928; https://doi:10.1001/jama.2021.5333

2   Wandell BA, Le RK. Diagnosing the neural circuitry of
    reading. *Neuron* 2017; 96:298–311; https://doi.org/
    10.1016/j.neuron.2017.08.007 (open access).
3   Taraskevich PS, Gibbs D, Schmued L, Orkand RK.
    Excitatory effects of cholinergic, adrenergic and
    glutaminergic agonists on a buccal muscle of *Aplysia*.
    Developmental Neurobiology 1977; 8:325–335; https://doi
    .org/10.1002/neu.480080405.

APPENDIX: THE MIND DIET BASICS

In 2015, the MIND diet (Mediterranean–DASH Intervention for Neurodegenerative Delay) was introduced specifically to target slowing of cognitive deterioration, both in normal aging and in Alzheimer's disease. The MIND diet combines most elements of the Mediterranean and DASH diets while adding greater emphasis on green-leafy vegetables, beans, nuts and berries. The components of the MIND diet are shown below, along with recommended servings for both the brain-healthy and brain-unhealthy food groups.

Ten brain-healthy food groups are:

Green leafy vegetables (kale, collard, spinach, salad)	6 or more servings/week
Other vegetables	1 or more servings/day
Nuts	5 or more servings/week
Berries	2 or more servings/week
Beans	4 or more servings/week
Whole grains	3 or more servings/day
Fish (not fried)	1 or more servings/week
Poultry (not fried)	2 or more servings/week
Olive oil	Primary oil used
Wine (optional)	1 glass/day

Five brain-unhealthy food groups are:

Red meats (includes beef, lamb, pork and ham)	Less than 4 servings/week
Butter and stick margarine	Less than 1 tablespoon/day
Cheese	Less than one serving/week
Pastries and sweets	Less than 5 servings/week
Fast fried food	Less than once per week

Media sources for more information:

www.mayoclinic.org/healthy-lifestyle/nutrition-and-
healthy-eating/in-depth/improve-brain-health-with-the-
mind-diet/art-20454746
www.today.com/health/mind-diet-plan-foods-eat-what-
mind-diet-t183797

Clinical Trials

Finding a trial doesn't have to be hard. If you or a loved one has Alzheimer's or is at risk for Alzheimer's, and you are interested in learning more about volunteering for a study near you, visit the Alzheimer's Association TrialMatch webpage: https://www.alz.org/alzheimers-dementia/research_ progress/clinical-trials/trialmatch. For a more comprehensive list, see clinicaltrials.gov. In the UK, information about volunteering for a clinical trial can be found on the Alzheimer's Society webpage: www.alzheimers.org.uk/ research/get-involved.

RESOURCES

2022 Alzheimer's Association Facts and Figures. https://
www.alz.org/media/Documents/alzheimers-facts-and-
figures.pdf. This PDF is updated yearly and can be
downloaded at the link above. It is my go-to source for
information about Alzheimer's and the related dementias.
It is completely up to date and thorough, but it is also accessible to the general reader.

Books

These books offer valuable contributions to the Alzheimer's literature and to the effort to raise awareness of the
medical, social and intimate dimensions of Alzheimer's
disease and the Alzheimer's experience.

Lynn Casteel Harper, *On Vanishing: Mortality, Dementia,
and What It Means to Disappear* (Catapult, 2020). The author
draws from her professional experience as a chaplain and
from art, literature and media coverage to discuss how society deals with aging and Alzheimer's. She shares some
case stories that exemplify the best and worst of Alzheimer's care, most from patients with late-stage Alzheimer's,
including her grandfather.

Lisa Genova, *Still Alice* (iUniverse, 2007). Dr. Lisa Genova is
a neuroscientist whose grandmother had Alzheimer's disease. Her first novel is the story of a psychology professor
in her fifties who begins to have memory loss and disorien-
tation. It is a gripping novel, seen through the professor's
eyes and the eyes of her family as she rapidly progresses

through early-onset, autosomal-dominant Alzheimer's. I read it in 2009 before I had any idea that I would have Alzheimer's, and it made a profound effect on the way I understood and interacted with my dementia patients.

Joseph Jebelli, *In Pursuit of Memory: The Fight Against Alzheimer's* (Little, Brown & Company, 2017). This is another book by a young neuroscientist. His grandfather died of Alzheimer's, and he does research in the field. It is a substantive, nonfiction history of Alzheimer's disease, from the story of Dr. Alois Alzheimer's first discoveries, to a number of individual personal stories of people with the disease, to a survey of current knowledge and research.

Jason Karlawish, *The Problem with Alzheimer's: How Science, Culture and Politics Turned a Rare Disease into a Crisis and What We Can Do About It* (St. Martin's Press, 2021). Dr. Karlawish is a professor and co-director of the Penn Memory Center at the University of Pennsylvania. This book is comprehensive yet accessible, covering the history, politics, and controversies surrounding Alzheimer's disease. It is thorough and it is compassionate. I highly recommend it.

Lauren Kessler, *Dancing with Rose: Finding Life in the Land of Alzheimer's* (Penguin Books, 2007). After her mother died of Alzheimer's, Kessler, who teaches nonfiction writing at the University of Washington, immersed herself in the world of dementia care by working for six months in an entry-level job at a local Memory Care facility. This is not an exposé of the nursing home industry. It is more about the lessons that she learned about getting close to people with advanced dementia and appreciating not only what they have lost, but what they still retain and what they have to offer. She begins to understand the relationship she had, or in some cases failed to have, with her own mother. This is an important and touching book.

Wendy Mitchell, *Somebody I Used to Know: A Memoir* (Ballantine Books, 2018). Chronicling her struggle with early-onset Alzheimer's, the author, after a career in the British health service, turns her efforts to ways to slow her cognitive decline and to help inform others about the challenges and opportunities in living with Alzheimer's.

Greg O'Brien, *On Pluto: Inside the Mind of Alzheimer's: New Horizons Expanded Edition* (Codfish Press, 2018). Greg O'Brien is a journalist who first developed signs of Alzheimer's after a head injury in his fifties. He writes eloquently about his experiences with the disease, first caring for his parents, who both had Alzheimer's, and then about his own battle. Greg is a friend, and appears in *Tattoo*.

Gerda Saunders, *Memory's Last Breath: Field Notes on My Dementia* (Hachette Books, 2017). A former university professor, Saunders takes a down-to-earth approach to her annotated life with dementia, and finds rich veins of memory to explore from her childhood in South Africa.

David Snowdon, *Aging with Grace: What the Nun Study Teaches Us About Leading Longer, Healthier, and More Meaningful Lives* (Bantam Books, 2001). Written nearly twenty years ago, this longitudinal study of several hundred nuns as they aged transformed much of the thinking about Alzheimer's disease and still is a fascinating read.

INDEX